REDUCING CHILD MALTREATMENT

Treatment Manuals for Practitioners

DAVID H. BARLOW, *Editor*

Recent Volumes

REDUCING CHILD MALTREATMENT

A Guidebook for Parent Services

JOHN R. LUTZKER
KATHRYN M. BIGELOW

Series Editor's Note by David H. Barlow

Foreword by David A. Wolfe

THE GUILFORD PRESS
New York   London

47837900

3-27-02

© 2002 The Guilford Press
A Division of Guilford Publications, Inc.
72 Spring Street, New York, NY 10012
www.guilford.com

Printed in the United States of America

This book is printed on acid-free paper.

Last digit is print number: 9 8 7 6 5 4 3 2 1

Library of Congress Cataloging-in-Publication Data

Lutzker, John R., 1947–
    Reducing child maltreatment: a guidebook for parent services / John R. Lutzker,
Kathryn M. Bigelow; foreword by David A. Wolfe.
        p. ; cm. — (Treatment manuals for practitioners)
    Includes bibliographical references and index.
    ISBN 1-57230-704-8 (pbk.)
    1. Child abuse—Prevention.   2. Family services.   I. Bigelow, Kathryn M.   II. Title.   III. Series.
    [DNLM: 1. Child Abuse—prevention & control—United States.   2. Family Therapy—
United States.   3. Parent–Child Relations—United States.   4. Parenting—psychology—United States.
WA 320 L9749r 2001]
RC569.5.C55 L88 2001
616.85′822305—dc21

                                                                                                2001040936

About the Authors

John R. Lutzker, PhD (University of Kansas), is Chief of the Prevention Development and Evaluation Branch of the Division of Violence Prevention, National Center for Injury Prevention and Control, Centers for Disease Control and Prevention. At the time this book was written, he was the Florence and Louis Ross Distinguished Professor and Chair of the Department of Psychology and Director of Graduate Training in Behavioral Psychology at the University of Judaism. He previously served as Acting Provost of the University of Judaism. He is also an adjunct professor of human development at the University of Kansas.

Dr. Lutzker is a past Editor of *the Behavior Therapist* and the *APA Division 25 Recorder*. He has been Associate Editor of *Education and Treatment of Children* and is currently on the editorial boards of the *Journal of Family Violence*, the *Journal of Behavior Therapy and Experimental Psychiatry*, *Child and Family Behavior Therapy*, *Behavioral Interventions*, the *Journal of Developmental and Physical Disabilities*, and *Children's Services: Social Policy, Research, and Practice*. Dr. Lutzker is the author of *Behavior Change* (with Jerry Martin) and *Ecobehavioral Family Interventions in Developmental Disabilities* (with Randy V. Campbell) and editor of the *Handbook of Child Abuse Research and Treatment*.

Kathryn M. Bigelow, MA (University of Kansas), is a doctoral candidate in developmental and child psychology in the Department of Human Development and Family Life at the University of Kansas. Her research interests are in violence prevention and parent–child and caregiver–child interactions.

Series Editor's Note

Empirical support appears weekly on the development of powerful and precise psychological treatments. In study after study, these new psychological features provide additional benefit to the "common" factors exercised by any skilled clinician, which include promoting meaningful relationships and instilling hope. Although these efforts have been well documented for adults, it is a largely overlooked fact that the psychological treatments for problems arising in children or in the context of families are among the strongest in our armamentarium of interventions. Now, John Lutzker and Kathryn Bigelow provide us with an excellent and important resource for intervening with families that maltreat their children. Among the problems encountered by psychologists, few are more tragic than families presenting for treatment who profess to love their children but who inflict harm and suffering on them in some way. This is not an uncommon presentation. As Lutzker and Bigelow point out, child protective service agencies in the United States in 1996 investigated more than 2 million reports of maltreatment of more than 3 million children and substantiated at least 1 million of these reports. This represents an 18% increase from 1990. Maltreatment in this sense involves both neglect and physical abuse. Almost 80% of the perpetrators are parents. The comprehensive assessment and treatment programs described in this book have been evaluated in the context of providing service to more than 1,500 maltreating families. Furthermore, this program, based on the ecobehavioral model, goes beyond reducing maltreatment and incorporates procedures that facilitate the development of a healthy and clean environment. Any child or family clinician or individual involved in creating health care policy for children should become familiar with this program, which should be disseminated widely.

DAVID H. BARLOW

Foreword

Some days it seems that we have not come very far in addressing the fundamental causes of child abuse and neglect, much less in preventing them. The problem seems as serious as ever, and the complex list of contributing causes—poverty, inequality, adherence to corporal punishment, to name but a few—have remained largely unchanged over the past several decades. Given our current inability to address this problem effectively, we may wonder if child maltreatment simply coexists within a culture that has forgotten its priorities and lost its collective compassion for disadvantaged members of the community. The news is not all bad, however. Increased efforts by clinicians, researchers, government planners, and child welfare advocates over the past two decades have made encouraging progress in tackling some of the fundamental causes of child abuse and neglect. Laws have been passed, funds have been allocated for detection, treatment, and prevention, and every community in North America is aware of the problem and is searching for ways to help maltreated children and their families. The time is ripe to provide communities and families with the information, resources, and skills they require to raise their children in a safe and caring environment.

The present volume is rich in clinical wisdom and reflects extensive experience in assisting families with multiple and complex difficulties that often surface in the form of child maltreatment. Due to the often adversarial nature of the program, parents who have come to the attention of child protective services have often lost sight of their most important role: to cultivate a protective, supportive, and nurturing relationship with their children. The authors of this guidebook show us many of the valuable ways that we can work with maltreating parents and their children to make their lives more rewarding and to reduce the risk of harm. For those of us seeking ways to reduce child maltreatment and promote healthy family relationships, the authors offer guidance and suggestions, rather than "solutions."

Project 12-Ways (and its replica, Project SafeCare) was the early product of an "eco-behavioral" approach to working with multiproblem families, which emphasized comprehensive services to assist parents in a manner that best approximates their natural environment. The detailed explanations, examples, case studies, intervention procedures, and data collection tools contained in this guidebook taught me a great deal about the different approaches we can take to assist families in a meaningful way. While not a substitute for training and experience, the ideas and methods presented herein are an invaluable resource to those of us seeking innovative, child- and family-focused ways to address the universal problem of child maltreatment.

For over 20 years John Lutzker and his colleagues have supported their view that working with maltreating families requires flexibility, a breadth of knowledge, and intensive in-home services. They have demonstrated that, despite the number of significant obstacles, children and youth who have experienced abuse or neglect can make major shifts in how they relate to others, especially if treatment is well matched to each family's unique circumstances and needs. As the field of child maltreatment develops from one of detection to one of prevention and assistance, this guidebook undoubtedly will provide important steps for many to follow.

DAVID A. WOLFE, PhD, ABPP
Professor of Psychology and Psychiatry
The University of Western Ontario

Preface

Child maltreatment is widespread. The National Incidence Studies (National Center on Child Abuse and Neglect, 1993) have shown that its prevalence has increased. All states in the United States have child maltreatment reporting laws and services. The federal and state governments mandate and fund services, and many privately funded organizations also provide services. Many of these services are no doubt very good. The problem, as often noted in the professional literature in child maltreatment, is that there exists very little and, in general, very poor evaluation of child maltreatment services. Further, there are few empirical studies demonstrating the efficacy of given programs or procedures. There are large, well-funded programs that have many site replications, yet it is rarely known how closely the services may resemble each other. That is, there is a problem known as fidelity, or lack of integrity of the independent variable. This means that although a staff member may be "trained" to provide a given service protocol or protocols, there are no direct observations or measures taken to ensure that the protocols taught are being delivered correctly.

This book comes out of a need to describe procedures that are valid and on which measures of the integrity of the independent variable have been done. The work presented here stems from more than 20 years of professionally validating, revalidating, and replicating the protocols presented here. Thus this book can serve not only as a resource but also, importantly, as a manual for other professionals to replicate these service protocols in their work in trying to treat the perpetrators of child maltreatment. In no way is this effort considered a panacea, but we do know that these procedures can be very effective in giving skills to parents. This book is primarily intended as a manual for professionals who may wish to apply the programs described herein. It could also be used as a supplementary text in classes dealing with parent training or other similar social services.

In Chapter 1 we define child maltreatment, provide evidence of its incidence and prevalence, detail the professional history of the field, and briefly describe the kinds of services that have been offered by the professional community. The chapter also reviews the ecobehavioral model from which the procedures described in this book were developed and validated. Chapter 2 describes Project 12-Ways, the first ecobehavioral program aimed at the treatment and prevention of child maltreatment. It also sets forth Project SafeCare, the replication of Project 12-Ways, and the effort that directly produced the protocols described here. The chapter also details the evaluation tools we feel are essential in examining the outcome of these procedures or the programs in which these procedures may be used. The recommended research designs reflect our bias toward understanding the individual more than understanding the group. Additionally covered in this chapter is program evaluation, a necessary component of any service project.

Chapter 3 offers an overview of the assessment and treatment services detailed in the rest of this book. This chapter again reflects our bias toward assessment that focuses on operationally defined behaviors that can be directly observed. We recommend some standardized indirect assessments that we have found useful as well. An overview of all assessments and treatments, and how these fit into 19 sessions, is provided. We also offer recommendations of additional treatments that can be provided to child victims of maltreatment. Professionals should be prepared to refer families whom they are seeing for counseling and other services.

Chapter 4 presents detailed procedures for assessing parent bonding skills. The protocols for teaching bonding skills through Planned Activities Training (PAT) and Parent–Child Interaction (PCI) training are reviewed in detail in Chapter 5. We have tested this approach on a number of participant populations, especially families involved in child maltreatment. We have found it extraordinarily effective for giving nonpunitive child behavior management skills to parents. This issue is particularly sensitive when working with families involved in child maltreatment.

Home safety is the focus of Chapter 6. The Home Accident Prevention Inventory—Revised (HAPI-R) is detailed, along with protocols for teaching parents how to make their homes safer for their children. Many families are referred to child protective services because of the unsafe conditions of their homes. Thus this safety program provides professionals with assessment and behavior change skills to improve these conditions for those families.

Chapter 7 provides the protocols for teaching parents child health care skills. We provide checklists that list the supplies that parents should have on hand, quizzes for parents to take on child health care, health care scenarios for parents to practice, and protocols for teaching these skills.

Staff training is the focus of Chapter 8. The bias that we show here is again on the teaching and measurement of skills, in this case for staff. We provide a hands-on model for staff training and describe how to monitor and maintain skills once training has terminated. The chapter ends with a summary and our conclusions about offering the services covered in this book.

Naming people to whom we would like to give credit for helping us with this book is risky because so many have helped in various ways over the years. In particular, all of the staff of Project 12-Ways in Illinois from 1979 to 1985 and the staff of Project SafeCare in California from 1994 to 1998 were instrumental in helping us create, evaluate, and provide these services. In particular, we acknowledge the assistance of Dr. Maria Lynn Kessler and Hilary Taub for their assistance in the development of the health and safety protocols. Nealdenea De Jesus has been helpful in conducting some of the final follow-up in assessing Project

SafeCare. Randi Sherman provided endless assistance in helping us with manuscripts and was the office manager for Project SafeCare. Gerald Hitsman also provided help with the manuscript, Barbara Watkins of The Guilford Press rendered invaluable editorial assistance, and Adam Cohen assisted in the preparation of the indices. The staff and administrators for the San Fernando Valley Department of Child and Family Services and the Valley Presbyterian Hospital Maternity Center deserve our thanks for their assistance and cooperation in identifying families who would benefit from being involved in the project and for their ongoing support and involvement. Finally, very special thanks are due to our families, who provide constant support and encouragement.

Project SafeCare was funded by a grant from The California Wellness Foundation (TCWF). Created in 1992 as a private and independent foundation, TCWF's mission is to improve the health of the people of California through proactive support of health promotion and disease prevention programs.

Contents

1

Child Maltreatment
and the Ecobehavioral Model

Few of society's problems are so puzzling and of such concern as child maltreatment. Why would adults, especially parents, intentionally inflict injury on a child? Why would parents neglect a child's basic needs? It is also surprising that, although child maltreatment has occurred throughout human history, it was officially recognized by professionals in the United States only in 1962, when Kempe, Silverman, Steele, Droegemueller, and Silver published their seminal article on the "battered child syndrome." In fact, it is well documented that the first successfully prosecuted case of child maltreatment in the United States was done so through the Society for the Prevention of Cruelty to Animals in the late 1800s, because at that time there were no laws protecting children.

Despite this "late" attention to the problem, considerable progress was made in the second half of the twentieth century in the development of theory, assessment tools, empirically derived treatments, and outcome evaluation (Lutzker, 1998).

DEFINITIONS OF CHILD MALTREATMENT

The problem of child maltreatment poses rather unique definitional issues. The actual act of physical or sexual child abuse is seldom directly observed. Neglect, in particular, is difficult to see because it is generally considered to be a problem of omission. It represents the lack of various caregiving behaviors, the omission of which causes harm or even death to a child. Like abuse, it is primarily a problem measured by various outcomes.

The National Research Council (NRC; 1993) reviewed the problem of defining child maltreatment and made a number of recommendations. First, they recognized that there are four generally accepted categories of child maltreatment: physical abuse, sexual abuse, neglect, and emotional abuse. This book focuses on physical abuse and neglect.

Subcategories of child maltreatment also need to be considered when formulating definitions. These are the following: endangerment versus demonstrable harm; the severity of the acts; the frequency of the acts; the class of potential perpetrators; the intent to harm and the culpability of the perpetrator; the developmental level of the child; and culturally informed definitions.

Child maltreatment can be identified in medical settings or through reports to child protection agencies. Reports to agencies often come from schools, but they can also come from a variety of other sources.

Legal definitions form a basis for defining child maltreatment, but they are still wanting for an empirical base (Portwood, Reppucci, & Mitchell, 1998). It has also been pointed out that part of the problem of defining child maltreatment is the lack of clear empirically derived standards of acceptable parenting (Greene & Killili, 1998).

Thus, in the context of the ongoing debate as to how best to define child maltreatment, for our purposes in this book we regard physical child abuse and child neglect as a function of referrals received from child protective services for those problems. In general, those agencies still regard abuse as an act of commission on a child by which physical harm has been perpetrated and neglect as the omission of safe and healthy provision of care to a child.

INCIDENCE

In 1996, child protective service agencies investigated more than 2 million reports of the maltreatment of more than 3 million children (U.S. Department of Health and Human Services, 1995). Nearly 1 million of these reports were substantiated; this was an 18% increase in an 6-year period from 1990. Thus the national rate of victimization was 15 per 1,000 children. Fifty-two percent of these children were the victims of neglect; 24% were the victims of physical abuse. Seventy-seven percent of perpetrators were parents. Thus programs that focus on parent training and other services are of particular relevance in the provision of services.

The most common victims of physical and emotional abuse are toddlers, preschool children, and young adolescents. Neglect is most commonly reported with very young children, that is, infants and toddlers. The incidence rate for child maltreatment is much higher for families of low socioeconomic status (SES) than for other SES groups (Wolfe, 1999). Also, children living with single parents are at higher risk for maltreatment than children living in two-parent households.

HOW CHILD MALTREATMENT AFFECTS ITS VICTIMS

There are many negative sequelae for the victims of child maltreatment. Many of these negative side effects are seen during childhood, but they can also be seen in adult victims of child maltreatment. For example, Wolfe (1999) notes that children who are victims of child maltreatment often fail to develop trust, have received little affection from others, and have had only highly authoritarian parenting styles modeled for them. Thus, as adults, these individuals may have considerable difficulties in relationships. These adults are also prone to other psychiatric problems. They are three times more likely to suffer mood disorders and two to four times more likely to suffer from an anxiety disorder. Violent and antisocial behavior is also common for victims of child maltreatment.

As children, victims of child maltreatment are at risk for lagging behind their age-mates in cognitive and social development. There is evidence of problematic attachment in children who are victims of child maltreatment. Wolfe (1999) has also noted that these children may have difficulty in inferring and understanding the intentions of others, thus causing problematic interactions with peers and eventually dating problems.

Academic performance and IQ have been shown to be affected by child maltreatment. A 20-point difference in IQ was seen in preschoolers who were victims (Hoffman-Plotkin & Twentyman, 1984). Abused children are significantly more aggressive toward peers and "show a complex array of social behaviors indicative of poor self-control, distractibility, and negative emotion, such as low enthusiasm and resistance to directions" (Wolfe, 1999).

Thus being the victim of child maltreatment leaves a child prone to many negative effects and often leads to serious problems in adolescence and adulthood. This fact behooves us all the more to create effective programs to intervene in and prevent child maltreatment.

PARENT CHARACTERISTICS

For years, it has been documented that there are some common demographic characteristics of parents who maltreat their children. These parents typically are single parents or have unstable adult–adult partnerships. Children in these families are also often born in very close succession. Poverty, parenthood at a young age, social isolation, and unrealistic expectations about child development are all factors that have also been associated with maltreating parents. Another major factor is substance abuse, thought to occur in the majority of abusing parents. Mothers are more commonly reported for neglect (90%) than are fathers. Spouse abuse is highly correlated with child maltreatment.

HISTORY

In earlier times, much of everyday life included what we would regard today as child maltreatment. In more difficult economic times, children were forced into harsh labor. This situation, of course, still prevails today in many countries. American companies have been accused of perpetuating child labor abuses in other countries, even though there are laws in the United States forbidding it. The State of Pennsylvania ran up against the religious and cultural practices of some of its own citizens when the state challenged some Amish communities who were employing their own children in their community industries. Because Amish people do not use modern industrial equipment, their children are put to work in production in their plants. They also have a cultural belief that these practices are necessarily developmental for their children. In this case, we can see how history, culture, and definition all play a role in the way child maltreatment is viewed.

As mentioned earlier, professional attention was first paid to child maltreatment in the

United States in 1962. That makes the field a very young one in the history of human services. The field is also probably more multidisciplinary in nature than most human service fields. This characteristic is both useful and problematic at the same time. It is useful in that the many disciplines that often work together to address child maltreatment each have something significant to offer. Each discipline thus can learn much from the others. The dilemma is that each discipline has different ways of conducting research and providing intervention services. Each also has differing theoretical underpinnings. Coordination is not always simple. However, the field will remain multidisciplinary, and thus each field must continue to work with the others to establish theory, research, and practice.

THEORIES OF CHILD MALTREATMENT

The field of child maltreatment has been lacking a well-established and recognized theory. Shortly after the professional recognition of the problem in 1962, the earliest theories were largely psychodynamic in nature and looked inward to the individual perpetrator in order to try to help explain child maltreatment. These theories never gained much acceptance and had not been researched with maltreating families.

Subsequently, social–ecological theories evolved. Belsky (1980) was the first to suggest a social–ecological perspective in child maltreatment. Others (Wolfe, 1987) followed with refined and expanded models. These examined the context of child maltreatment, suggesting that the phenomenon was a function of several mitigating social–ecological factors, such as parental unemployment, poverty, substance abuse, poor parenting practices and personal histories of childhood maltreatment, and certain child characteristics, such as having a disability or displaying challenging behaviors. Although research supports these social–ecological theories, they have two primary deficiencies. The first is that the observations of the factors that appear related to child maltreatment do not account for the numerous families in similar circumstances who do not maltreat their children. The second is that they do not account for cognitive factors, such as the expectations parents have about children in general and their own child in particular, or for the attributions that parents make about their children's behavior.

A comprehensive theory of child maltreatment should thus consider social–ecological factors and cognitive elements. Azar and her colleagues (Azar, Povilaitis, Lauretti, & Pouquette, 1998) have proposed a metamodel of child maltreatment, taking several important factors into account. They point out that models to explain child maltreatment have differed on many dimensions, such as definitions, assumptions, levels of analysis, complexity, and model form. Among the assumptions that have tried to explain child maltreatment have been defect, deficiency, and disruption models, explained in the following.

In defect models, the problem is assumed to be caused by a parental or child defect that cannot be corrected. This kind of model does not offer hope for any successful amelioration of the phenomenon.

A deficiency model suggests that the parent lacks adequate parenting skills. This assumption allows that a parent can be taught new skills to help overcome child maltreatment.

The disruption assumption suggests that environmental factors are key in creating child maltreatment. Although there is evidence that factors such as poverty play a role in the problem, the existence of many families who live in abject circumstances and who do not engage in child maltreatment argues against disruption as the sole mitigating factor in child maltreatment. Finally, others have made assumptions that there are differences or mismatches between typical modes of responding and the inappropriate modes displayed by maltreating families.

Taking some of these assumptions into account, Azar and her colleagues have suggested that an integrated metamodel should include factors that are amenable to change and that intervention should also allow for prosthetic strategies. Such a model must take into account parent-based cognitive disturbances and behavioral skills deficits. These are examples of factors that would be amenable to change. Azar et al. (1998) also suggest that child developmental factors be an integral part of theory and treatment. Thus parent training and child treatment relevant to a 5-year-old child victim of abuse would not be the same as for a 9-year-old victim.

The five domains that Azar et al. (1998) recommend be considered in a metatheory are cognitive disturbances, parenting skill problems, impulse control problems, stress management deficits, and social skills problems. There are skill training and treatment programs that have been demonstrably effective in dealing with these factors. Several of the chapters in this book offer protocols for dealing with some of these factors.

RATIONALE FOR THE ECOBEHAVIORAL MODEL

The rationale for the ecobehavioral perspective is, as Azar has suggested, that the models are as good as the ability to affect change from them. Thus if social–ecological factors play a role in child maltreatment, along with cognitive and biological factors, then it seems only logical that treatment services should try to affect skill building and behavior change protocols that influence a family's social ecology such that the further risk of child maltreatment is reduced.

The ecobehavioral model evolved from a series of articles that were published in the *Journal of Applied Behavior Analysis* in the 1970s. The journal had published a dialogue between ecological psychologists and applied behavior analysts in which the ecological psychologists suggested to the behavior analysts that they needed to examine child behavior from a broader perspective. The ecological psychologists lauded the behaviorists for their focus on the direct observation of behavior and their empirical approach, but they cajoled them into looking additionally at behavior in broader context and looking at how changing the behavior of a child at home or in school might subsequently affect that child's social ecology. From those discussions came the term "ecobehavioral." The first description of the ecobehavioral approach to prevention and intervention in child maltreatment was offered by Lutzker, Frame, and Rice (1982) in their description of Project 12-Ways, discussed later in this book. They took an ecobehavioral perspective that resembled what Azar et al. (1998) have called for in looking at the many factors that may mitigate child maltreatment. Thus, as we describe, data are collected in a variety of settings, and intervention services represent a broad range of offerings related to skill deficits in parents that may contribute to their social ecologies and produce child maltreatment or that may put the children in the families at risk for maltreatment.

DEFINING "ECOBEHAVIORAL"

What is meant by "ecobehavioral"? Breaking the word up helps explain it. The "eco" in "ecobehavioral" refers to a philosophy and practice of viewing problems such as childhood maltreatment from a social–ecological perspective. This means that there is an attempt to assess and treat the family's social ecology rather than to view child maltreatment as a psychiatric problem of the parent or as a simple risk problem for the child. Thus, for example, data from direct observations and from some standardized measures on the child, the parent, parent–child interactions, others in the child's social ecology such as siblings, the school, teacher–child interactions, and the home environment (such as safety hazards, discussed in Chapter 5) should be collected. Other settings might be assessed, for instance, parent–child interactions in several community settings, such as the grocery store, the shopping mall, or the playground.

The "behavioral" part of "ecobehavioral" refers to the direct assessment of skills and behaviors and to the use of direct intervention and training strategies such as those that are described in subsequent chapters. In other words, although insight-oriented strategies may be useful with some psychiatric disorders and some life crises, in child maltreatment the ecobehavioral approach focuses on the direct teaching of skills that help change the individual's social ecology such that the child is put at lowered risk for maltreatment. Thus, for example, direct skills, such as parent training and/or stress reduction, are taught to families. Increasing skills that maltreating parents lack reduces the risk of maltreatment of their children in the future.

In addition to viewing the family as a social ecology and to teaching skills, several pieces make up the ecobehavioral approach. First, all ecobehavioral services are delivered to families *in situ, never* in a clinic or office setting. That is, parent training is conducted in the home and in the community. Stress reduction training is conducted in the home. Needless to say, home safety training is conducted in the home, along with health training. The reason for the *in situ* delivery of ecobehavioral services is that conducting teaching and training in this manner increases the likelihood of generalization of the skills.

Generalization is sought, or should be, in any intervention service, across time, behaviors, and settings. By across time, we are referring to the durability or maintenance of treatment. Thus we can expect newly learned skills to be displayed over time when those skills have been taught in the natural setting. Similarly, previous research has demonstrated (Huynen, Lutzker, Bigelow, Touchette, & Campbell, 1996) that providing planned activities training to parents in their homes produces generalization of the parenting skills and improvements in child behavior in many community settings in which those skills might not have been directly trained. Finally, we have also routinely seen that parents are able to generalize the skills they have been taught with one child to other children in the family and that parents show generalization by displaying the skills they have been taught with different challenging behaviors that the child may display.

EFFECTIVE PROGRAMS FOR TREATING CHILD MALTREATMENT

Chapter 2 describes in detail the programs on which this book is based—Project 12-Ways and Project SafeCare. Here we mention some other programs that have, like ours, an empirical bent and that have been effective in providing intervention and prevention services in child maltreatment. For example, Hansen and his colleagues (Hansen, Warner-Rogers, & Hecht, 1998) described a program called FISP (Family Interaction Skills Project). This was a multi-faceted ecobehavioral approach to families who had been referred for child maltreatment. It included a comprehensive assessment package largely utilizing direct behavioral assessment techniques similar to those we describe in Chapter 3. Families received systematic parent training, and training in problem solving, home safety, hygiene, budgeting skills, nutrition, and several other related skills. Outcome measures showed considerable success for this program as it was delivered to families in rural West Virginia.

Fantuzzo, Weiss, and Coolahan (1998) described a model of integrating community members in developing and carrying out a program. They were interested in improving the social skills of poor children who had been the victims of abuse. Child victims of abuse often lag behind their developmental age-mates in a number of skills, including social behavior. Of particular note in the work of Fantuzzo and his colleagues was their use of community members in the inner-city 100% African American sample with whom they worked to help develop the assessment protocols and implement the treatment program.

The community members stressed that they wanted assessment to focus on skill development rather than skill deficits, and the researchers thus incorporated this component into the design of the assessment (based on direct observation of the children's behavior). A play-buddy system was used whereby preschool peers with good social skills were taught how to teach social skills to the abuse victims. Community members were also recruited to help promote generalization of the skills in the classroom. This research provides a fine model of incorporating the community into research and service.

Striefel, Robinson, and Truhn (1998) have described a wraparound service for families at risk or involved in child maltreatment in rural Utah. They developed a program called the Community–Family Partnership (CFP), which provides and coordinates a number of services for families. Their needs assessment addresses employment; housing; financial management; physical, dental, and mental health; family functioning; parenting skills; social self-sufficiency; homemaking skills; transportation; public assistance; and a transition plan for leaving the CFP. Some of these services are provided directly by the CFP; others are referred.

Outcome measures from the CFP have suggested considerable improvements in areas in which the families displayed initial deficits. These services have been provided to a wide range of poor people in rural Utah.

Holistic injury prevention has been the focus of the work of Peterson and Gable (1998). They have noted that so-called unintentional injury to children merely represents a continuum of some form of parental neglect in most cases. They believe that most injuries are preventable. Children in families involved in child maltreatment have far more injuries than children in families not reported for abuse or neglect. Thus Peterson and her colleagues have suggested a variety of approaches for preventing injury and maltreatment. Parent training is a primary focus of their approach. Additionally, they have suggested that a correct understanding of developmental levels of children and of expectations about child behavior are very important variables to teach parents. Knowing a child's limitations or what behavioral expectations are reasonable at different ages is critical in injury prevention.

Peterson and her colleagues suggest that parents must be knowledgeable about children's impulse control (or lack thereof), about the child's ability to take perspectives, and about developmental triggers. Further, parents must be taught to adequately supervise their children and not to rely on rules that the children may not be prone to follow but rather to set up safe environments for their children. Additionally, parents must learn to control their own anger, must receive help if they are depressed, and must learn nurturing skills if they do not already display them.

A culturally sensitive violence-prevention program for African American children and adolescents was described by Yung and Hammond (1998). This school-based program teaches such social skills as how to receive negative feedback and how to negotiate. Faulty cognitive responses, such as believing that victims do not suffer, and hostile intentions are reviewed, and more adaptive cognitive responses are taught. Additional components of the program include education in violence risk, reinforcement systems, and environmental features and the use of language familiar to the children and adolescents. Extensive facilitator training is a key component of the program.

Direct observation of skills, ratings of behavior, and school records form the outcome measures for this program. Self-ratings, school records, and juvenile court records have all indicated success in preventing violence through this program.

Another adolescent prevention program, the Youth Relationships Project (YRP), has shown similar success in Canada. The YRP also uses cognitive–behavioral strategies to teach adolescents violence prevention (Pittman, Wolfe, & Wekerle, 1998). Outcome data from this project have also been encouraging.

Parents with intellectual disabilities have been the focus of the work of Feldman (1998). These parents are at especially high risk of maltreating their children. Feldman has used pictorial cues as training tools to teach a variety of child care skills to these parents. Feeding, hair washing, sleep safety, bottle cleaning, nutrition, crib safety, diapering, bathing, and treating diaper rash have been taught through the cue technique. Parents who receive this training are able to demonstrate skills equal to those of parents who do not have intellectual deficits. Tymchuk (1998) has developed a similar program and has also demonstrated that parents with limited intellects are quite capable of learning basic child care skills if given the proper training.

Projects 12-Ways and SafeCare, discussed in Chapter 2, have shown parent training to be a useful approach to families involved in child maltreatment. In Chapters 4 and 5, we detail our parent training model, based on an ecobehavioral perspective. Many families are referred to child protective service agencies because of the unsafe or unclean conditions in their homes. In fact, the most common child maltreatment referral is for neglect, frequently environmental neglect. Chapter 6 details our home safety intervention program. Teaching health care skills is an important aspect of services to families referred for child maltreatment. Chapter 7 describes our protocols for teaching young parents child health care skills. Most experts who have provided services to families involved in child maltreatment agree that these families often become chronic cases within the child protective service system because of their problem-solving deficits. Thus, in Chapter 3, we describe protocols for teaching problem-solving skills. Also described in that chapter are recommendations for teaching child safety skills, the direct treatment of the child as related to anxiety and other behavior problems that often surface as a result of maltreatment, and the need to refer parents for depression counseling. To provide services to families experiencing multiple stressors and problems, it is essential to be aware of the variety of resources available in the community. A model for staff training, suggestions for staff meeting format, multicultural issues, and addressing setbacks are discussed in Chapter 8.

2

The Ecobehavioral Model in Action: Project 12-Ways and Project SafeCare

The development of the services presented in this book began with Project 12-Ways in 1979. The services were refined and the findings systematically replicated in Project SafeCare. The history of both projects, the evolution of the services, and the outcome research are reviewed in this chapter.

PROJECT 12-WAYS

An application of the ecobehavioral model, Project 12-Ways was initiated on July 1, 1979, as a federally funded Title XX contract between the Illinois Department of Children and Family Services and the Behavior Analysis and Therapy Program of the Rehabilitation Institute at Southern Illinois University. Since then, the project has expended millions of dollars, serving more than 1,500 families and training hundreds of students and professionals in the ecobehavioral model for child maltreatment. Operating also out of universities, the model has been replicated in West Virginia, Nebraska, Mexico, Florida, and California. It has been disseminated through professional publications and dozens of research and discussion articles. In the process, publications have addressed individual behavior change in families by sharing case studies and single-case experiments, and research has been conducted with several families showing the efficacy of one service component or another. Program evaluation data have consistently shown that families served by Project 12-Ways are at lower risk for recidivism during and after treatment than matched comparison families who are also involved with child protective service agencies and who receive services other than Project 12-Ways in the same region. Project 12-Ways is a true application of the ecobehavioral model. It is *in situ* and provides multifaceted assessment and services.

The model was derived from then-budding social–ecological theories. At that time, however, treatment, especially empirically driven treatment, for child maltreatment was very limited. Early case studies reported some successful use of simple parent training or stress reduction. Both of those approaches seemed to make some sense as techniques to help physical child abuse perpetrators gain skills to prevent further incidents; however, they also seemed too simple to durably change some of the factors that may have led to the child abuse or neglect for which the parent had been reported.

Treatment Services of Project 12-Ways

In writing the proposal for Project 12-Ways, we considered several factors that had been associated with child maltreatment in proposing an ecobehavioral assessment and treatment model. The initial 12 services, all intended to be delivered *in situ*, were: parent–child training, stress reduction, self-control training for parents, basic skills training for children, activity planning, reciprocity (relationship) counseling, alcoholism referral, job finding, money management, health and safety training, multiple-setting behavior management, and prevention.

Parent Training

The rationale for parent–child training seemed simple. If, in fact, there were deficiencies in many perpetrators' behavior management skills, then teaching simple behavior management skills would seem a logical intervention. Further, because some studies had shown the value of stress reduction training, it would seem especially reasonable to combine this type of training with parent training. Parent training can be cumbersome and demanding. The parent is asked to be consistent in applying a program involving procedures that may seem awkward, especially when the parent may be facing everyday stressors that make the follow-through of newly learned behavior management techniques difficult to employ. For example, a young mother may be worried about mounting bills that she has no resources to pay and may be concerned that her boyfriend, who recently left her and stole her food stamps, may return and cause further difficulties for her. In the presence of such stressors, it may be very difficult to apply consistent parent training unless the parent is provided with some actual skills, such as progressive muscle relaxation or behavioral relaxation training (Poppen, 1988). Thus the rationale for the ecobehavioral model became one of combining training in several types of skills aimed at changing some of the factors that appear to contribute to child maltreatment.

Self-Control Training

Self-control training for parents focused on anger management. Teaching children basic self-control skills was a function of the data that suggested that child victims of physical abuse and neglect lag behind their age-mates in developmental skills. Thus teaching children basic hygiene or toileting skills might help reduce their direct risks. Further, we learned that teaching these skills directly to the children impressed their parents that we had something to offer and helped us proceed with services such as parent training, with which the parents were more cooperative after they had seen us teach something to their children.

Activity Planning

Activity planning was instituted because so many families involved in maltreatment seemed to lack the everyday activities and schedules of families not involved in child maltreatment. This component of Project 12-Ways has evolved into Planned Activities Training (PAT), an active component of our current services that is described in detail in Chapter 4.

Reciprocity Training

Although conducted on a limited basis, reciprocity training was used to help adults (parents and their spouses or partners) to get along better with each other, something that again the literature has suggested as a frequent deficiency in adults involved in child maltreatment. An example of this kind of counseling was described by Campbell, O'Brien, Bickett, and Lutzker (1983), who used reciprocity in combination with parent training and stress reduction to treat a self-referred mother who had migraine headaches and was concerned that she would kill her child if she did not receive assistance. Reciprocity marital counseling was instituted with the woman and her husband after stress reduction had been successful at lessening her headaches and after parent training had improved her child behavior management skills.

Alcoholism Referral

Many perpetrators of child maltreatment abuse substances. In such cases, referral to alcohol and drug abuse programs is essential in programs such as Project 12-Ways.

Job Finding

Unemployment and underemployment are factors associated with child maltreatment. Thus helping parents find jobs, if they are interested, makes eminent sense from an ecobehavioral perspective. In addition to the economic benefits of employment, having a job improves self-esteem, may improve a perpetrator's relationships with significant others, and allows the perpetrator less time spent in the home with children. Presuming appropriate child care, less time spent in the home with the children can be beneficial, allowing the parent to spend better quality time with his or her children.

A very well-regarded job-finding program is the Job-Club (Azrin & Besalel, 1980). Although highly successful, the Job-Club does involve a group effort by job seekers, often a problem because of the insular nature of the families that were seen by Project 12-Ways. An individualized version of the Job-Club was developed whereby the Project 12-Ways counselor helped the parent specify job goals, look at job advertisements, write a resume, network and schedule interviews, and practice interviews. Many poor mothers in rural southern Illinois are trapped by the fact that working at a low-paying job often creates more of a financial bind than staying at home to care for the children and accepting public assistance.

Money Management

Being poor and often having educational and problem-solving deficits causes money management to be a frequent problem for families involved in child maltreatment. Thus money management skills should be taught to these families. Often money management requires simple systems, such as savings envelopes that have pictures of the savings goal on them. For example, when a paycheck or public assistance check arrives and is cashed, the counselor can help the parent put some cash in an envelope for the utility bill, for example, by putting a picture of an electric light bulb on the envelope. These families often found themselves without money for Christmas gifts and would spend all of their money in December on gifts, often leaving them with no money for food, rent, and other important bills. We have used envelopes with pictures of Christmas trees so that the parents can put aside a few cents each week for holiday gifts.

Economic stress can often lead to situations that put children at higher risk for abuse. Thus learning some basic money management skills can help the parent avoid these risk situations.

Health and Safety Training

Neglect is the most common reason for child maltreatment referral. Neglect often involves unsafe and unhealthy living conditions in the home. Thus we have developed an assessment tool, the Home Accident Prevention Inventory—Revised (HAPI-R; Mandel, Bigelow, & Lutzker, 1998), and the Checklist of Living Environments to Assess Neglect (CLEAN; Watson-Perczel, Lutzker, Greene, & McGimpsey, 1988). Each of these validated assessment tools allows service providers to quantify health and safety hazards in homes. Changing these conditions can be accomplished through the techniques that we recommend in Chapter 5.

Multiple-Setting Behavior Management

The term "multiple-setting behavior management," originally articulated in Project 12-Ways, simply meant that the services were delivered *in situ*. Delivering services in the natural setting has several advantages. First, there is a lower risk of attrition. Families involved in child maltreatment are not prone to show up at clinics, university centers, or other outside appointments. The ecobehavioral model involves delivering service in the natural environment. Not only does this increase the likelihood that the service will be delivered, but it also increases the likelihood that the service will be durable and that the parents and children will generalize the skills that they have learned. For example, we have had a number of parents tell us that, although they learned to use PAT with the child who was the reported victim of the abuse, they also successfully applied PAT to all of the children in the home. Parents also regularly report using the skills that they are taught in the home in community settings. In fact, we have research data to back up these reports (Huynen, Lutzker, Bigelow, Touchette, & Campbell, 1996).

Prevention

Prevention was the final component originally delivered in Project 12-Ways. This component involved teaching young parents a host of prenatal and postnatal skills, such as diet and health care during pregnancy and child health care after the delivery of the child. Chapter 7 describes many of these skills.

Conclusion

The strong features of Project 12-Ways notwithstanding, there are features that suggest further examination. For example, mental health and child protective workers have asked if the model can be implemented in mental health centers and by caseworkers when a university-based program such as Project 12-Ways is not available.

Project 12-Ways is also labor intensive and relatively cumbersome. Thus it would be productive to examine means for delivering these ecobehavioral services in a more efficient manner. Also, Project 12-Ways serves a primarily rural environment of mostly white families. How well could this service be replicated in an urban environment with other than white families? And what cultural issues present themselves in different regions with other than white families? These are some of the issues that produced Project SafeCare. The next section reviews our replication of Project 12-Ways, Project SafeCare, in which this dissemination/replication issue was partly examined.

PROJECT SAFECARE

Project SafeCare was what is known as a *systematic replication* of Project 12-Ways. This means that much of the model is the same but that there are some systemic differences between the two projects. Project SafeCare was funded by The California Wellness Foundation (TCWF) to address some of the concerns about Project 12-Ways. Specifically, we were interested in knowing if some of the services offered by Project 12-Ways could be delivered in a succinct fashion and if other sources of service delivery than graduate students could be effective. In order to keep the service delivery succinct in Project SafeCare, we chose bonding, safety, and health as the service components, based on a belief that these were the most important components that we could offer. Project SafeCare was to be delivered in an urban setting, as opposed to the rural setting of Project 12-Ways. Also, the research and graduate assistants from Project SafeCare would come from many universities around southern California, as opposed to the very specialized nature of the graduate program in southern Illinois. Further, the families served by Project SafeCare would be largely Latinos and Latinas from Mexico and Central America, a very different cultural group from the families served by Project 12-Ways in rural southern Illinois. We were also interested in assessing the outcome of Project SafeCare through direct observation assessments, as we did with Project 12-Ways, but also with some indirect assessment tools that are well respected in psychology and other social services. These tools are described in Chapter 3.

Types of Families Served

Two types of families were referred to Project SafeCare. One group consisted of families referred by the child protective service agency who had been reported and investigated for child abuse or child neglect. The other group consisted of families who were referred from a local hospital's maternal health education office. These families were considered at high risk for child maltreatment because the parents were young, mostly single, and poor. A social worker at the hospital had judged them to need the services offered by Project SafeCare.

After referral, Project SafeCare contacted families, and an initial meeting at the family's home was arranged. At the first meeting, the counselor explained the services offered by Project SafeCare to the family. They were introduced to and signed an informed consent form, and they were told that at the end of services they would receive a $25 grocery scrip coupon.

Forty-one percent of the families were monolingual Spanish speakers. Thus Project SafeCare employed fluent Spanish-speaking staff members. All manuals and materials provided and described in subsequent chapters were available in Spanish.

The most frequent order in which services were provided was: health care training, home safety, and Planned Activities Training (PAT). Prior to services, we assessed the families with an extensive demographic questionnaire and with a number of standardized tools. Those of primary interest were the Beck Depression Inventory (BDI; Beck & Steer, 1993), the Parenting Stress Index (PSI; Abidin, 1990), and the Child Abuse Potential Inventory (CAPI; Milner, 1986, 1994). Thus we used three types of assessment of the families: demographic questionnaire data; direct observation of home safety hazards, health care skills, and parent–child interactions; and indirect, standardized assessments (the three mentioned previously).

Intervention Services

Project SafeCare offered bonding, health care, and safety services, described in the bulk of the remainder of this book. These were three of the most common services provided by Project 12-Ways; each was modified for Project SafeCare in a systematic manner. By systematically modified, we mean that we conducted expert validation on each component and modified each component according to the results of the expert validation. These validations are explained in greater detail later in this chapter. As one example, for the safety assessment, we added balconies and water hazards that had previously been missing from the Project 12-Ways safety assessment.

It was logical to keep the safety skills training component in the services provided to Project SafeCare families. We had had previous success with the Home Accident Prevention Inventory (HAPI) as a tool to formally, yet easily and directly, assess the presence of home hazards accessible to children. It was necessary to revise and revalidate the HAPI; thus we tested the Home Accident Prevention Inventory—Revised (HAPI-R) with the families served by Project SafeCare. We also explored the use of video as a tool for reducing home hazards.

Evaluating the Efficacy of Project SafeCare

It is very important to formally address some larger questions about a project's effectiveness through program evaluation (Lutzker, 2000). During and after services, we used substantiated incidents of abuse and neglect as our primary measure of the effectiveness of the program. The term "recidivism" describes this. We used code numbers for the families involved so that after we were no longer involved with serving a family, we would not know the names of subsequent perpetrators; but we do know how many families are found to score as recidivism cases.

Several program evaluations have been conducted on Project 12-Ways and Project SafeCare (e.g., Lutzker & Rice, 1987; Gershater-Molko, Lutzker, & Wesch, in press). In all cases we have found that families who received intervention services from either of these projects were less likely to show recidivism than matched comparison families. That is, we compared families served by Projects 12-Ways and SafeCare with families who were identified and case-managed out of the same child protective service offices. These comparison families were referred by the child protective services to services other than Project 12-Ways or Project SafeCare. In each evaluation, it was found that the comparison families had statistically higher recidivism rates than the Project 12-Ways or Project SafeCare families. Lutzker and Rice (1987) looked at 5 years' worth of follow-up data. In four of the five yearly comparisons of more than 350 families in each group, recidivism rates ranged from 6 to 14% lower for Project 12-Ways than for the comparison families. Gershater-Molko, Lutzker, and Wesch (in press) examined survival rates of Project SafeCare families. They found that 85% of Project SafeCare families had no reports of child maltreatment 2 years after terminating services. Only 56% of the comparison group had "survived," that is, had no reports during the same period. In another program evaluation with Project 12-Ways, it was found that the comparison families had a shorter history with the child protective service agencies than the Project 12-Ways families (Wesch & Lutzker, 1991). The caseworkers from child protective service agencies had frequently reported that they referred their most difficult cases to Project 12-Ways. Thus one might consider the longer histories with the agency prior to referral of the Project 12-Ways families as a measure of severity. That is, it might be concluded that the Project 12-Ways families, who, in fact, had better outcomes than the comparison families, were also more severe cases to begin with. This strengthens all the more the conclusion about the overall efficacy of the project. For Project SafeCare, the data after 2 years showed that families who received services were significantly less likely to be reported again than the comparison families. Because these results replicate the recidivism program evaluation data from Project 12-Ways, we feel comfortable in suggesting that the ecobehavioral model is more effective at reducing child maltreatment risk than other services often mandated by children's protective service agencies.

Finally, another kind of program evaluation we have used is social validation (Wolf, 1978). This is a process by which consumers of a service are asked about their perceptions of the goals, processes, and outcomes of the services. We used this process to ask questions of agencies with which we work.

To conduct a social validation program evaluation, we ask questions about whether or not the goals set for the consumer were appropriate; for example, whether the interventions were themselves practical, easy to learn, handled professionally, and so on. The consumer answers by rating effectiveness on a Likert scale. The questions are presented on a survey that is left with the consumer or agency respondent to fill out when the project personnel are not present. Leaving self-addressed stamped envelopes with the respondent helps increase the return rate, along with assurances of anonymity. From this kind of feedback, grouped data can suggest how happy or unhappy consumers are with services, and the program can be adjusted accordingly. For example, O'Brien, Lutzker, and Campbell (1993) found that all services of their project were rated satisfactorily, with the exception of staff's knowledge about legal issues pertaining to the consumers. From this feedback, workshops were then conducted to improve the staff's knowledge about these issues.

In addition to asking these kinds of questions directly of consumers, we recommend asking them about agency personnel, particularly pertaining to the professionalism of the staff. Thus agencies who work with the project can be asked not only about the goals, processes, and outcomes of the services as the agency perceives these with regard to the consumers served but also about whether the staff are timely, professional, and knowledgeable.

Table 2.1 shows some sample questions from social validation evaluations.

We thus strongly recommend these kinds of assessments of intervention programs. Additionally, cost–benefit analyses can be conducted as a kind of program evaluation, although these kinds of analyses are often cumbersome and inconclusive.

Several intervention components of Project SafeCare have been evaluated using the strategies we have addressed here. For example, the use of video as a teaching tool to reduce home safety hazards in two families was demonstrated through a multiple baseline design across settings (i.e., different rooms in each home; Mandel et al., 1998). After baseline data were collected in each home, video was introduced sequentially in different rooms. For example, in the first family, after video training was successful in reducing safety hazards in the living room, it was used to reduce hazards in the bathroom. After changes were seen in the bathroom, the bedroom safety video was shown. Finally, after safety hazards were reduced in the bedroom, the kitchen video was shown, and similar success occurred. Thus internal validity of the intervention (video) is demonstrated when behavior change occurs after the sequential introduction of the intervention.

Both the case-study approach and single-case research design were used to report considerable improvements and to evaluate the Spanish Project SafeCare protocols with a family (Cordon, Lutzker, Bigelow, & Doctor, 1998). The case-study method was used to show dramatic improvements in the child health care skills of the mother. During baseline assessment, the mother demonstrated only 25–50% of the required skills. After practice with the protocols described in Chapter 7 of this book, the mother showed 100% performance at a 5-month follow-up observation.

With this same family, a multiple-baseline design across settings was used to show that PAT was effective in improving parent–child interactions. Finally, a multiple baseline across rooms showed that direct home safety instruction by the Spanish-speaking staff caused significant reductions in the number of safety hazards accessible to the children in the home.

A multiple-baseline design across participants (parents) was used to show the effectiveness of video in teaching PAT skills (Bigelow & Lutzker, 1998). The video was first shown to one parent. After her skills improved considerably, the PAT videos were shown to the second

TABLE 2.1. Sample Social Validation Questions

Outcome questions

Health Care Training

1. Caring for my child's health when he or she is not ill has become easier.
2. Recognizing that my child is ill has become easier.
3. Knowing when to take my child to the doctor has become easier.
4. It has become easier to recognize when my child needs emergency treatment.
5. As a result of this program, I am more confident that I am better prepared to care for my child when he or she is sick.

Home Accident Training Program

1. Since I have completed the safety program my home is. . . .
2. Conducting the safety program in other homes where small children live would be. . . .
3. I am better able to identify safety hazards in my home.
4. While having the individual who conducted the safety training program look through my home, I was. . . .
5. How much time did it take to make your home safe for children?

Parent–Child Interaction Training Program

1 The Parent–Child Interaction Program has improved my relationship with my child.
2. I feel more patience toward my child.
3. I enjoy the time I spend with my child more.
4. My child's behavior has not improved.
5. I would recommend the Parent–Child Interaction Program to other parents.

Procedure questions

Rate how useful each of these items was in helping you benefit from the services you received, if relevant.

1. Counselor's explanations
2. Counselor's demonstrations
3. Practicing during sessions

Staff questions

The counselor who conducted the safety training program . . .

1. Was warm and friendly.
2. Was helpful.
3. Gave clear explanations.

Video questions

If you observed Project SafeCare's video during training, please respond to the following statements: The videotapes . . .

1. Were easy to understand.
2. Were useful and informative.
3. Contained too much information.

Agency questions

1. Staff from Project _____ returned my phone calls in a timely manner.
2. Staff from Project _____ were knowledgeable about our agency's regulations regarding services.
3. Staff from Project _____ were helpful and cooperative at meetings.

parent, who also demonstrated considerable improvements. Finally, multiple baselines across health care skills were used to show that a research assistant, a caseworker, and a nurse could each be successful in teaching these skills to families (Bigelow & Lutzker, 2000).

Information on recidivism rates and recipients' social validation give an overall picture of program success. More specific evaluation methods, such as direct observation, were used to measure specific aspects of the program.

Content Validation of Direct Measures

Although indirect measures, such as standardized tests, were used for assessment evaluation in Project SafeCare, direct measures, such as recording the number of hazards in a home or the number of steps on a checklist of parenting skills, were the primary measures. Because some of the direct measures were designed specifically for use with the Project SafeCare teaching components, they had not necessarily been as thoroughly evaluated as standardized questionnaires, such as the CAP-I, PSI, or BDI. Before conducting any assessments with families, a content validation of these measures was conducted.

The home safety assessment device, the HAPI-R, was an extension of the Home Accident Prevention Inventory (HAPI; Tertinger, Greene, & Lutzker, 1984). This measure was revised from its original version to include hazards that were commonly present in the urban area in which Project SafeCare took place (see Mandel et al., 1998, for an additional description of this validation). A search of the most common reasons for serious childhood injury or death indicated that, in addition to the categories represented on the HAPI, children are at risk for injury or death from falling and drowning hazards. In Los Angeles, California, where many families live in apartment buildings with balconies and possibly poorly maintained door latches and locks, this finding was especially relevant. Definitions of these categories were devised, and then operational definitions for every type of hazard represented on the HAPI (along with the new categories of hazards) and the measurement strategies were sent to home safety professionals. They were asked to rate each type of hazard for its importance in ensuring a safe home for young children. From their ratings, the revised HAPI-R was finalized, ensuring that there was validity to this assessment device.

The behaviors observed during parent–child interaction training were also subjected to content validation (see also Bigelow & Lutzker, 1998). The operational definitions of the parent–child interaction skills (which are described in detail in Chapter 5) were sent to 17 experts in child development. The experts were asked to rate the importance of assessing each of the behaviors when evaluating the quality of the parent–child relationship. These professionals included teachers, child care directors, clinicians, and researchers. Eleven of these individuals returned their completed surveys. Each respondent was asked to rate the importance of measuring each behavior when assessing the quality of the parent–child relationship. If 75% of the respondents reported that a given behavior was important or essential (a 4 or 5 on a 5-point Likert scale), the behavior was included in the assessment protocol. If fewer than 75% of the respondents reported that a behavior was important or essential, it was not included. None of the behaviors were rated in this manner, however. Additional suggestions and questions provided by the respondents were addressed by revising the existing behavioral definitions. Thus the operational definitions for the behaviors assessed when evaluating parent–child interactions were based on the validation provided by objective child development experts.

In the health training component, the contents of the symptom guide, of the Health Recording Chart, and of a list of recommended medical supplies that should be in homes were validated by 11 physicians and family practice medical residents (see Bigelow & Lutzker, 2000, for an additional description). The items in the symptom guide, which functioned as a medical reference guide for parents, were revised according to feedback provided by the physicians and residents. As with the parent–child interaction validation, if 75% of the respondents rated an item as a 4 or 5 on a 5-point scale of importance (with 5 being "essential"), the item was included in the guide. These same criteria were used in revising the Health Recording Chart and the list of recommended medical supplies.

One additional form of validation used in the evaluation of the home safety training component was expert outcome validation (Mandel et al., 1998). Several photos of various areas in the home in which hazards were found, such as the kitchen counter or the couch in the living room, were taken both at baseline and at posttraining in the homes of two families. These photos were presented in random order to children's social workers from the referring agency. The pictures were unlabeled; thus social workers were unaware of which pictures were taken at baseline and which were taken at posttraining. The social workers were asked to rate the overall safety of the areas depicted in each photo on a 3-point scale. Although the pictures did not depict areas as clearly and in such detail as they might be if the social workers had seen them in person, they provided an indicator of the general condition of the home. For each area, the social workers rated the areas in the posttraining pictures as safer than those in the baseline pictures.

Thus these additional forms of validation—content validation and, in the case of home safety training, expert outcome validation—provide support for the use of these measures. Feedback and guidance received from experts in the areas of home safety, child health care, and parent–child interactions were used to refine our procedures and to lend validation to these measures, which were designed for use with the training components. Data from these direct measures were then used for evaluating specific aspects of the program.

Looking More Closely at How Project SafeCare Works

Program evaluations, such as the use of social validation questionnaires and the comparison of recidivism rates with other programs, showed the overall efficacy of Project SafeCare. Program evaluation, however, is only one of five ways in which Project 12-Ways and Project SafeCare were evaluated. These methods can be used with any program of similar size. They are (1) clinical evaluation, (2) case studies, (3) single-case experiments, (4) multiple-participant research, and (5) program evaluation. This section discusses each in turn, ending with further kinds of program evaluation.

CLINICAL EVALUATION

The first method, at the simplest level, is what we call "clinical." By this we mean that collecting data on treatment variables is an extremely important aspect of empirically based ecobehavioral research and treatment. Thus data can be collected on variables such as the frequency with which a parent praises her child or the use of incidental teaching techniques. Staff members can sometimes collect these data; other times it may be possible to have the parents collect the data themselves. These "clinical" data are seldom if ever published; however, they are of considerable value and can be used for several purposes. First, they can be used to show progress or a lack of progress to a parent. Thus, for example, if the service provider is trying to help the parent increase his or her use of descriptive praise of the child's appropriate behavior, data collected by the provider during observations or by the parent, with some previously discussed definitions, can be examined. If baseline data are available, those data can be compared with intervention data. The parent can thus see the progress of the treatment program.

Clinical data can also be used for supervision. Again, although these data seldom meet any scientific criteria for use in published research or case studies, they are useful as a mechanism for staff–supervisor communication about the progress or lack thereof with a family being discussed in a supervision session. The data form a common ground for language between the supervisor and the interventionist. Thus, if an increase in the parents' use of descriptive praise is a goal, the data on this variable can be examined in graphic form by both the supervisor and staff member. Problem solving can occur if the data show a lack of positive progress. If the data show progress, the supervisor has an opportunity to praise the provider, and the two can decide what the intervention criteria should be and if it is time to move on to other components.

Clinical data were used in this very manner in Project SafeCare. Staff meetings always included a review of the clinical data for each family. In each meeting the data on bonding, health care skills, or safety were reviewed, and follow-up observations were scheduled that produced data 1 month, 2 months, and 6 months after the termination of intervention. The health care data and the safety data, in particular, were also reviewed with the family. A part of the home safety program is to show the family the number of hazards that are accessible, as demonstrated by observations made using the HAPI-R. The clinical data were most useful in serving staff and families in Project SafeCare.

CASE STUDIES

Another important way in which to evaluate and present information from a project such as SafeCare is through case studies. These are published reports of clinical information that are otherwise not publishable because the data do not meet more rigorous scientific criteria. Normally, to publish clinical data, at least two requirements must be fulfilled. These are that the data are reliable and that they have internal validity. By reliable it is meant that at least two observers have independently observed the behavior being recorded in at least 25% of the observation sessions. That is, each observer observes and records simultaneously, and their data are compared. The other criterion, internal validity, means that an acceptable research design has been used that allows the clinician, researcher, and the scientific community confidence that the changes seen in behavior are, in fact, a function of the independent variable (intervention) and not of some other events that may have occurred at the same time in the family's life. As anyone who has been involved in a human service project knows, it is not always possible or practical to conduct reliability observations or to be able to utilize a research design. These, however, are instances in which a case study can serve an important purpose in that it allows the creative researcher or clinician an opportunity to share an important innovation with the professional community.

Kazdin (1982) articulated when and how case studies are to be used. A case study is an example of a novel procedure or intervention that does not meet the scientific criteria just outlined but does show an innovative intervention when both dramatic behavior change of previously refractory behavior occurs *and* when the intervention procedures are described in sufficient detail to be easily replicated. When these case studies are published, they allow researchers to further examine the internal and external validity of the new intervention.

A case study from Project SafeCare was presented within the context of an article that also described additional research. In that report, Cordon and colleagues (1998) described the evaluation of a Spanish protocol for teaching health care skills to a monolingual Spanish-speaking mother who was referred because of physical abuse of her 6-year-old son. The baseline assessment, through direct observation of the skills that are described in Chapter 7, indicated that this mother had few of the requisite skills for identifying illnesses and determining whether the illness could be treated at home or whether the child should be taken to the physician. As shown in Figure 2.1, she, in fact, correctly displayed only 25–50% of the skills.

After the baseline assessment, the mother was given written materials describing how to conduct the protocols for identifying and reporting illnesses. Figure 2.1 shows, as was the case for almost all parents given only written materials, that her skill level did not improve. Thus the mother was provided five sessions of hands-on practice of the protocols. After that training, as can also be seen in Figure 2.1, the mother displayed 100% of the skills by the sixth

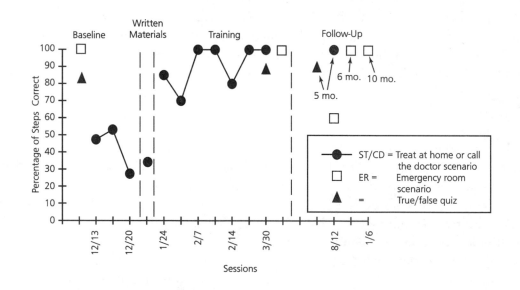

FIGURE 2.1. Percentage of steps correctly followed by parent on a health-parent behavior checklist using three types of health scenarios (treat at home, call the physician, and emergency treatment) and percentage of correctly answered items on a 10-item true–false health quiz. From Cordon, Lutzker, Bigelow, and Doctor (1998). Copyright 1998 by Elsevier Science. Reprinted by permission.

observation session. It was also very important that, when observations were made 5, 6, and 10 months following the end of training, this mother had maintained her child health care skills.

This is a good example of the utility of a case study. There is no research design for this presentation. The baseline condition was followed by the written materials condition, which was, in turn, followed by the training. Nonetheless, the data show clear and dramatic change in important skill development with this parent who had been reported for child maltreatment. Sharing this information in a scientific journal allows other researchers to further evaluate the protocol. The case study also confirms a consistent result that we have found over the years: Hands-on training is virtually always superior to relying on written materials to teach skills.

SINGLE-CASE EXPERIMENTS

The Cordon et al. (1998) report also represents a single-case experiment, the next level of sophistication in evaluating a program such as Project SafeCare. A single-case experiment makes use of a robust single-case research design with one family or individual. Additionally, directly observed and measured data are reliable in that a second observer has independently recorded data, and agreement between the two observers is 85% or better. Figure 2.2 shows data from the single-case experiment with the same Spanish-speaking family. The figure represents data collected during observations of parent–child interactions prior to, during, and after training in PAT. Three training settings were measured in which the parent interacted with the child during play, while dressing the child, and during bath time. A generalization setting, mealtime, was chosen to see if the mother also demonstrated the skills she had learned in the other three settings without having receiving training during meals. As can be seen in Figure 2.2, before learning PAT, her appropriate parenting skills (which are explicated in Chapter 4) occurred only 55–60% of the time during playtime, 60% percent of the time while dressing the child, and around 75% of the time during bath time. During meals she demonstrated the requisite skills from 50% to 75% of the time. After learning PAT, her skills were at 100% in all settings, including meals, meaning that this mother showed generalization in an untrained situation. Even 5 months after training the skills had been maintained nicely.

Reliability data between two observers was 85%. Thus this report represents a single-case experiment in that there were reliably collected data, there was a research design known as a multiple baseline across settings, and the research was conducted with just one family. The multiple-baseline design shows that it was PAT that was responsible for the change in the parent's skills and not some other events that occurred in this family during the same time because skill levels showed improvements only after training occurred in PAT sequentially over time.

The single-case experiment provides scientifically valid information about the efficacy of a treatment such as PAT. It lacks external validity in that we cannot say that this would work with other families served by the project or those served elsewhere. But sharing these data allows for possible replications and thus for the demonstration of external validity, the confidence that the training has generality.

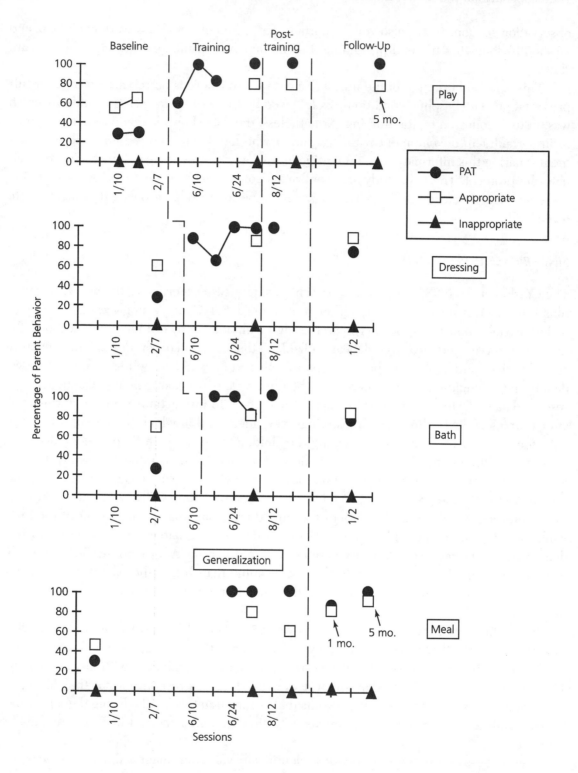

FIGURE 2.2. Percentage of appropriate and inappropriate parent behaviors on a Parent–Child Interaction data sheet and percentage of steps correctly followed by parent on a PAT checklist in four daily living activities. From Cordon, Lutzker, Bigelow, and Doctor (1998). Copyright 1998 by Elsevier Science. Reprinted by permission.

MULTIPLE-PARTICIPANT RESEARCH

Research with more than one family or participant is the next level of evaluation. An example of this type of research was a study conducted with two Project SafeCare families who had been reported for child abuse (Bigelow & Lutzker, 1998). In one family the mother was the perpetrator; in the other family it was the father. Video was the training mode for PAT in these two families. Figure 2.3 shows the parenting skills during baseline and after video training. This is a multiple-baseline design across families, showing that video was, in fact, responsible for the improvements in parenting skills, because the skills improved only when the video was introduced sequentially across time.

Another example of research from Project SafeCare involved the teaching of health care skills across a number of families (Bigelow & Lutzker, 2000). In this case a number of single-case replications showed that hands-on training of health care skills resulted in criterion performances by the young parents who were taught to identify and report or to treat their children's illnesses themselves. In this research, research assistants, caseworkers, and a nurse all demonstrated that they could successfully train young parents in child health care skills. Training involved teaching the parents to follow a series of steps to identify symptoms, to use reference and record-keeping materials, to determine the best form of treatment, and to either treat the illness at home, consult medical personnel, or seek emergency treatment. These skills were assessed through direct observation of the parents in simulated health care

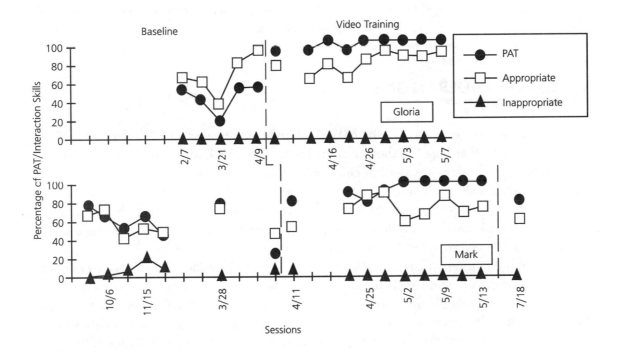

FIGURE 2.3. Percentage of appropriate and inappropriate parent behaviors as scored on a Parent–Child Interaction data sheet and percentage of steps correctly followed by parent on a PAT checklist for two parents. From Bigelow and Lutzker (1998). Copyright 1998 by Haworth Press, Inc. Reprinted by permission.

scenarios. A series of multiple-baseline designs across parents showed the effectiveness of the training protocols.

PROGRAM EVALUATION

Program evaluation—asking larger questions about the overall effectiveness of a project—represents the final level of assessment and evaluation that should occur in any research and service effort. Project SafeCare has addressed several questions of program evaluation. We discussed overall questions of recidivism and social validation earlier. Another method of evaluation was to examine the grouped data on the direct assessment measures. That is, we compared baseline and posttreatment data from families who completed all three Project SafeCare treatment programs, in safety, health, and bonding. We found statistically and clinically significant differences in all three areas. That is, the families showed very large reductions in the accessible hazards in their homes, the parents were able to demonstrate child health care skills, and there were significant improvements in the parents' use of PAT skills.

In addition to examining the grouped data from the directly observed behaviors, we also examined pre- and posttest differences in standardized indirect assessments. The "industry standards" in depression, parenting stress, and child abuse risk are the BDI (Beck & Steer, 1993), the PSI (Abidin, 1990), and the CAPI (Milner, 1986, 1994), respectively. We were very pleased to learn that there were clinically and statistically significant pre- and posttest differences in each of these measures. Thus, after receiving services from Project SafeCare, parents were less depressed, showed less parenting stress, and were at lower risk for future child maltreatment. These are very important results, and each measure correlates with the other.

OTHER CONSIDERATIONS

Why are these interventions effective? We think they are effective because families appreciate learning skills that improve their relationships with their children and, in some cases, because they help the families get the child protective service agencies "off their backs." We have conducted social validations that show that the families express satisfaction with the goals, process, and outcomes of the interventions. Additionally, those who have completed training have said that they would tell and have told friends and families about the interventions and have recommended the services to them.

Although the program has been clearly effective with those families who have completed the training, there are some considerations worth mentioning. Our attrition rates were high, as they are in all research and service projects dealing with child maltreatment. Some attrition is unavoidable, given the nature of the problem and some of the characteristics of maltreating families. One of the characteristics of these families is frequent relocation; they move often. These moves are often intended as an escape from the close eye of the child protective service agencies. Another reason for attrition could be assessment. We have suggested that assessments be kept to a minimum so that skill training can begin quickly. Offering quick training in this manner could cause some families to benefit sooner and so to stay with the intervention.

Although in our sample we employed fluent Spanish speakers as staff, there were still class differences between these staff and the families, the former being college educated. We have speculated that teaching parent graduates of our programs to provide the training to other parents may be a culturally sensitive way to reduce attrition.

It would have been very useful to collect emergency room data as another measure of the success of the safety and health components. However, in the densely populated urban area we served, our attempts to get accurate information from the more than 30 hospitals and clinics utilized by the families we served caused us to abandon the collection of those data.

In the next chapter we present an overview of the specific assessments and treatments we used in Project SafeCare.

3

Assessment and Treatment Overview

In this chapter we present an overview of the treatment services and related assessment procedures that are detailed in Chapters 4 through 7. We begin with an overview of treatment services. These include the three skills training areas tested in Project SafeCare, a review of additional services for which families can be referred, and a suggested course of treatment with logistics of delivery. In the second part of the chapter, we present an overview of assessment procedures; which include both direct observational techniques and indirect measures. Indirect measures are reviewed in this chapter. Direct assessment procedures, such as Planned Activities Training (PAT) and Parent–Child Interaction Training (PCI), are discussed beginning in Chapter 4. Other direct measures are described in detail with the respective skills training procedures.

AN OVERVIEW OF TREATMENT SERVICES

As reviewed briefly in Chapter 2, Project SafeCare found that services in three key areas were effective in reducing child maltreatment. These services are (1) bonding skills training; (2) home safety skills and cleanliness training; and (3) health care skills training. As this chapter explains, the assessment procedures are designed to identify deficits in these particular skills areas.

Bonding Skills Training

The bonding component consists of Parent–Child Interaction (PCI) or Parent–Infant Interaction training (PII). The primary technique for teaching bonding skills to young parents is Planned Activities Training (PAT). This training is described in detail in Chapter 5. PAT has been shown to be an effective approach in preventing challenging behavior and in producing effective and affective parent–child interactions in a variety of families who have children with a range of difficulties such as conduct disorder, autism, mental retardation, and attention-deficit/hyperactivity disorder (Huynen et al., 1996).

Until Project SafeCare, PAT had not been systematically evaluated with families involved in or at risk for child maltreatment. What makes PAT different from more traditional behavioral parent training approaches and thus useful for families involved in or at risk for child maltreatment is that it is aimed at preventing challenging behavior in children rather than reacting to challenging behavior with consequences. Thus PAT has built-in components that allow parents to incorporate them in all daily living and special activities. The incidental teaching component, described in more detail in Chapter 4, teaches parents to always act as teachers in increasing their children's use of language and in making every activity a learning one.

Safety Skills Training

Hazards that are accessible to children pose risks in any case and they are especially problematic in high-risk and child-maltreating families. Neglect is the most common reason for referral to a child protective service, and often in neglect situations home safety hazards play a role in the referral. The Home Accident Prevention Inventory—Revised (HAPI-R) was revalidated with the families served by Project SafeCare. The use of this inventory and the safety skills taught are described in Chapter 6.

Health Care Skills Training

The literature and experience clearly demonstrate that young parents need to learn how to care for the health needs of their children. Thus we revalidated the child health care skills training program we had developed in 1988. In doing so, we taught our Project SafeCare families a host of important child health care skills that had been validated by family practice physicians. These protocols are described in detail in Chapter 7.

Additional Services for Referral

Although the following services were not provided in Project SafeCare, it is important to consider that other services may be needed to address other problems or concerns within the family or may be of benefit to the family.

Problem-Solving Skills

Problem-solving skills are frequently deficient in parents involved in child maltreatment. That these parents often find themselves in repeated trouble with child protective service agencies is testimony to this skill deficit. Those working in the field of child maltreatment remain mystified as to why some of the same problems that continue to get the family into trouble persist. The family often seems to fail to learn from experience. Thus a young mother may repeatedly leave her young children alone at home when she goes out on dates, or that mother may continue to fail to budget money for her utility bill, leading to threats by the utility company to cut off her service. These kinds of problems seem amenable to problem-solving training.

Borck and Fawcett (1982) and others (MacMillan, Guevremont, & Hansen, 1988) have outlined systematic strategies for teaching problem-solving skills. The strategies involve providing assistance to help define the actual problem and then brainstorming with the individual in order to make a list of all possible solutions. Whether each potential solution is a good one is not judged. The individual is encouraged to list as many potential solutions as possible. Then, after this list is complete, each solution is evaluated. Pros, cons, overall feelings, and the availability of and requirements for each solution are listed. Then, based on this information, the individual can judge whether each solution is excellent, good, fair, or poor and then determine the best overall solution. This helps to clarify the problem and potential solutions. After a target date is set for beginning to implement the solution, the individual is also provided with assistance in taking steps to implement solutions, if necessary.

Child Safety Skills

Teaching children to be safe at home represents an underexplored area in child maltreatment research. No empirical studies have dealt with this important issue; thus, here, we are proposing that service providers and researchers consider the following. Children should be taught how to recognize the cues that may put them at risk for abuse. For example, if it is learned during assessment interviews that the child is at higher risk when the mother's boyfriend comes home drunk, then the child should be taught how to recognize this. The child can be taught through doll play, role play, or, better yet, video training. During this training the child could be taught to hide, play quietly, leave to a designated safe place, do chores, avoid the boyfriend, call 911, or any other response that will increase his or her safety.

Each of these safety skills, once identified, could be taught through simulation, role play, or video training, then the child could be asked to demonstrate the skills. The child would be given feedback on the correctly displayed skills and asked to practice those that may need additional work. The criterion for demonstrating mastery might be five consecutive role plays in which no errors were made.

Professionals in child maltreatment should validate the skills. Members of these professions should be sent surveys and asked what behaviors would be appropriate to include in such a child safety training protocol and in what situations these behaviors are appropriate. Items of common agreement taken from these surveys could then be placed in the protocol and taught to child victims of maltreatment.

Depression Counseling

Depression counseling is worth considering for parents, especially mothers, involved in child maltreatment. The literature has suggested that these mothers may display depressive symptoms. Of encouraging note, however, is the program evaluation data from Project SafeCare that suggest that levels of depression are statistically and clinically reduced in parents who receive Project SafeCare services. These data suggest that depression may be a function of having limited or lower skills in bonding, child health care, and home safety and that acquiring skills in these areas may reduce depression.

The BDI (Beck & Steer, 1993) is relatively simple to administer and score. It can be used to screen for depression or, as was done in Project SafeCare, to see if there are pre- or posttreatment changes in depression scores among treated families. Parents who maintain elevated BDI scores can be referred for treatment. The literature suggests that cognitive behavior therapy is the treatment of choice. A medical or psychiatric review should also accompany cognitive behavior therapy to determine if medication would be a useful adjunctive therapy.

Community Services

Awareness of community services is an important part of providing comprehensive services to families involved in child maltreatment. A family may be in need of any number of services or resources, such as depression counseling. Thus knowing what services are available to families is important in providing the services described in this book. Additional services that professionals serving families involved in child maltreatment should be aware of include: safe shelters for women and children; counseling services; ethnic counseling and recreational centers for the variety of ethnic groups in a given community; other recreational services; medical clinics; psychoeducational programs, such as parent groups; specialized groups, for example, for parents with children with medical or other disorders, such as asthma or autism; availability of local public transportation, housing resources, and advocates; child care resources; legal and immigration resources; local businesses; and city services. Having knowledge about the resources available in the family's neighborhood may also prove helpful. For example, knowing about the degree of safety in neighborhood parks, about the services provided by local churches, or about the activities offered through the local parks and recreation department may be crucial to helping the family obtain valuable resources that they might otherwise not have known existed. Finding out about local programs and services involves becoming aware of the surrounding neighborhoods in which families live and the local services that may be available.

OVERVIEW OF ASSESSMENT

A number of techniques can be used to assess parents, children, and family interactions in the context of child maltreatment. This section provides a description of the methods and instruments used in Project SafeCare to assess parent and child behavior, to guide interventions, and to evaluate the effects of the intervention. The assessment procedures reviewed here can also point to other skills or interventions that may be needed by parents, such as referral for depression counseling or training in problem-solving skills.

About Indirect and Direct Assessment Measures

Although some of the assessment measures used in Project SafeCare were used primarily for research purposes, these measures may also provide additional information that may be useful in conducting a thorough evaluation in order to provide more effective interventions. The measures used in Project SafeCare can be categorized into two categories: direct and indirect measures. Direct measures, which involve directly observing parent or child behavior, were the primary measures. Indirect measures consisted of standardized interviews or questionnaires.

Direct Assessments

The benefit of direct measures is that they allow the counselor to directly observe behavior rather than making inferences about behavior based on what parents or children tell us. Further, these measures are directly tied to the skills taught in each training component. For example, parents' health care skills were evaluated by calculating the percentage of steps the parent demonstrated correctly during a child health care scenario rather than by relying on parents' self-reports of how they might treat a childhood illness or injury. The specific measures used are described in the chapters that present each training component. Specific direct measures were designed for this program and their content validated, as discussed in the Chapter 2. The direct measures consisted of guidelines for the specific behaviors or skills to observe, together with checklists for recording observations during parent–child activities and interactions (bonding), for observing home safety and cleanliness conditions, and for parent knowledge and skills of infant and child health care. A description of these direct measures and how they are related to training may be found in Table 3.1. See also Lutzker, Bigelow, Doctor, Gershater, and Greene (1998) for an additional description of the measures used in Project SafeCare and Lutzker, Bigelow, Swenson, Doctor, and Kessler (1999) for a review of other assessment devices appropriate when working with families at risk for abuse and neglect.

In Project SafeCare, direct observation was an essential part of each training component. Direct observation data are collected before training begins, during each training session, and after training is completed. The data are used to assess changes in parents' and children's behavior and to evaluate the effectiveness of the training programs. Before training begins, data collected during direct observations inform the counselors of the areas in which the family needs assistance. These data, which are also collected throughout training, provide the counselor with evidence of the family's acquisition of new skills. For example, before beginning home safety training with a family, counselors conduct observations throughout the home to determine how many accessible hazards are present in each room. By knowing, for example, that there are 87 hazards in the kitchen, 43 hazards in the bathroom, and 5 hazards in the living room, the counselor is able to select the kitchen as the room most in need of childproofing. Immediately before each training session, counselors count the number of hazards present in each room in order to evaluate the effects of training. This information provides the counselor a valid and reliable means for determining when training is effective and when training is completed. If the number of hazards has not been reduced following training sessions in each room, the counselor and family then return to those rooms to address the remaining hazards. Follow-up observations are conducted at 1, 3, and 6 months following the completion of training. These observations provide additional information about the maintenance of these skills.

TABLE 3.1. Overview of Direct Assessment and Training Components

Infant and Child Health Care Skills

- Five training sessions
- *Objective*: Correctly identify symptoms of childhood illnesses or injuries and then determine whether to treat at home, consult a physician, or seek emergency treatment.
- *Direct assessment*
  - *Parent Behavior Checklist*. Record of steps completed correctly during role-play scenarios involving parents' treatment of childhood illnesses or injuries (see Appendix 7.7).
  - *True–false quizzes*. 10-item quizzes on general health knowledge
- *Skills taught*
  - Identify and record child's symptoms
  - Refer to health manual to determine course of treatment (treat at home, consult a physician, seek emergency treatment)
  - Treat children's illnesses
  - Take a temperature
  - Take a pulse
  - Give medications
  - Understand basics of good health
  - Get children immunized
  - Keep health records

Home Safety and Cleanliness Training

- Five training sessions
- *Objective*: Identify and eliminate accessible hazards, dirt, and clutter within the home.
- *Direct assessment*
  - *Home Safety: Home Accident Prevention Inventory-Revised (HAPI-R)*. Record the number of accessible hazards in eight categories of hazards within each room throughout the house.
  - *Cleanliness: Checklist for Living Environments to Assess Neglect (CLEAN)*. Record whether item areas are clean or dirty and the number of clothes, linens, and other items not belonging.
- *Skills taught*
  - Safety training
    - Identify accessible hazards within the home in eight categories of hazards
    - Determine the reach of a child and areas that are accessible to children
    - Make hazards inaccessible to children by placing hazards out of reach, in a locked container, or behind childproof latches
  - Cleanliness training
    - Understand three dimensions of cleanliness (clean and dirty, clothes and linens, items not belonging)
    - Learn general methods of cleaning
    - Identify areas needing cleaning
    - Implement methods of cleaning

Planned Activities Training and Parent–Child Interaction Training

- Five training sessions
- *Objective*: Provide engaging and stimulating activities for young children, thus preventing challenging child behaviors and increasing positive parent–child interactions.
- *Direct assessment*
  - *Daily Activities Checklist*. Ask parents to identify most challenging situations. When possible, most challenging situations are incorporated into training.

(continued)

TABLE 3.1. *(continued)*

- *PAT Checklists*. Assess use of strategies for preparing for activities in advance, engaging children in activities, and preventing challenging child behavior during play and daily routines, such as meals, dressing, or bath time.
- *Parent–Child Interaction Assessment*. Record the frequency of parent's and child's use of appropriate verbalizations and touch and parent's use of incidental teaching and instructions.

- *Skills taught*
  - Use positive interaction skills (attending, touching, communicating, instructing)
  - Identify difficult situations and settings
  - Prepare in advance for activities
  - Explain activities, rules, and consequences
  - Provide engaging activities
  - Use incidental teaching
  - Give choices
  - Ignore minor misbehavior
  - Give positive feedback and instructions for improving inappropriate behavior
  - Provide rewards or consequences

Indirect Measures

Indirect measures, such as interviews or questionnaires, provide a standardized method for assessing parent and child characteristics. These are used as a secondary measure and provide a standard that can be easily recognized and interpreted by researchers and clinicians. Further, when these measures are used to evaluate the effects of the intervention, the results can be compared with those obtained on other, similar projects. These measures are called "indirect" because they allow counselors to collect information about how people behave *indirectly*. They do not allow counselors to directly observe behavior, but they collect information that people report about their beliefs and behaviors. The indirect measures used in Project SafeCare were self-report measures and were administered to parents at baseline (pretraining), posttraining, and follow-up sessions. The disadvantage of these measures is that parents may misrepresent their responses, either purposefully or not (Hansen & MacMillan, 1990). The use of direct observation may compensate for this limitation. Direct observation strategies also have limitations, such as reactivity—that is, parents may "stage" their behavior because they know that they are being observed. For these reasons, both direct and indirect measures were used in Project SafeCare. We recommend a combination of both types. The indirect measures described here are a sample of the available measures that may be appropriate for families referred for abuse or neglect, who frequently experience multiple stressors and problems. Although these measures may be appropriate for many families, the selection of assessment measures should be based on the specifics of the child, family, and environment.

The direct measures used in Project SafeCare are described in detail in their respective chapters, so only indirect measures are described here. The manuals for these measures may be obtained from their respective publishers; they contain more thorough reviews of the research in which the measures have been used and evaluated. All parents completed the Child Abuse Potential Inventory (CAPI; Milner, 1986, 1994), the BDI (Beck & Steer, 1993), and the Parenting Stress Index (PSI; Abidin, 1990). See Table 3.2 for a review of these indirect measures.

TABLE 3.2. Indirect Assessments

Child Abuse Potential Inventory. Used to identify parents at risk for physical abuse of their child.

Beck Depression Inventory. Assesses the presence of depressive symptoms in adults.

Parenting Stress Index. Screens for family stress related to parent characteristics, child characteristics, and other situations that are directly related to the role of being a parent.

Parent Behavior Checklist (Fox, 1994). Identifies parenting strengths and needs related to expectations, discipline, and nurturing.

Parental Anger Inventory. Assesses anger experienced by abusing parents in response to challenging child behaviors.

Eyberg Child Behavior Inventory. Measures the frequency and intensity of children's disruptive behaviors.

Conners' Rating Scales. Assesses patterns of problem behavior related to conduct disorder.

CHILD ABUSE POTENTIAL INVENTORY (CAPI)

This 160-item measure is used to identify parents who engage in physical abuse toward their child. This instrument should be used as a screening instrument in conjunction with other assessment strategies and not as the sole measure of abuse potential (Milner, 1986, 1994). Parents report whether they agree or disagree with items falling into a number of domains. It is a widely used and researched measure of potential risk for physical abuse. This measure yields an Abuse Potential Score, as well as scores on six other scales: Rigidity, Unhappiness, Distress, Problems with Child and Self, Problems with Family, and Problems with Others. Cutoff scores for each of these scales are provided in the administration manual (Milner, 1986). There are also three distortion indices, which include Faking Good, Faking Bad, and Random Responding. These scores are derived from combinations of scores on three validity scales: Lie, Random Responding, and Inconsistency. The CAPI has a readability level of grade 3, making it appropriate for many parents. Evaluation of the CAPI has been extensive and has demonstrated support for its psychometric properties (see Milner, 1986, for the manual and Milner, 1994, or Milner, Murphy, Valle, & Toliver, 1999, for reviews). A Spanish version of the CAPI is available, although little research has been done on its use.

BECK DEPRESSION INVENTORY (BDI; BECK & STEER, 1993)

The BDI assesses the presence of depressive symptoms in adults and can be used to evaluate change in reports of depression following treatment. Depression can contribute to poor parenting practices or can be an outcome of poor parenting. Thus monitoring depression through a standardized assessment tool such as the BDI is prudent. Other depression assessments exist, but we use the BDI because it is well respected and easy to administer.

Twenty-one sets of four statements are included on the BDI. Parents read or are read a set of statements and then are asked to choose one of the four statements that best describes the way they have been feeling during the past week, including the current day. Items in each set are assigned a value of 0, 1, 2, or 3. The BDI score is obtained by summing the ratings given by the parent for each of the 21 sets. The maximum total score is 63. Scores falling between 10 and 16 may indicate mild depression. Scores between 17 and 29 indicate moderate depression, and scores above 30 may indicate severe depression. It is important, however, that an interview with a trained clinician is conducted to confirm the assessment.

PARENTING STRESS INDEX (PSI; LOYD & ABIDIN, 1985; ABIDIN, 1990)

The PSI was designed to screen and diagnose family stress that may increase the risk of dysfunctional parenting behaviors or behavior problems in the child. Three domains are assessed: parent characteristics, child characteristics, and other situations that are directly related to the role of being a parent (Abidin, 1990). The reliability of this measure has been demonstrated, supporting its use for both preliminary screening and evaluating the effectiveness of intervention. High scores on the Total Stress scale indicate that parents may be experiencing clinically significant levels of stress. High scores on the child characteristics domain are often associated with children who display qualities that are contributing to the overall stress in the parent–child system. For parents of children with disabilities (hyperactivity, mental retardation, cerebral palsy, emotional disturbances, learning disabilities, etc.), the child characteristics domain score is usually elevated above the parent characteristics domain (Loyd & Abidin, 1985). Additional research has supported the cross-cultural utility of a Spanish version of the PSI with Latina mothers (Solis & Abidin, 1991).

PARENT BEHAVIOR CHECKLIST (PBC; FOX, 1994)

This 100-item checklist can be used to identify parenting strengths and needs. The PBC is appropriate for parents of children aged 1 to 4 years and measures three aspects of parenting: expectations, discipline, and nurturing.

OTHER OPTIONAL MEASURES

Conducting all of the measures that follow with a family can be extremely time-consuming, taking away valuable time from teaching skills and providing support and assistance to families. Thus it is important to ensure that the measures used in assessment are appropriate for family members and that they will yield valuable information.

The Parental Anger Inventory (PAI; DeRoma & Hansen, 1994) was designed to assess anger experienced by abusing parents in response to challenging child behaviors. Parents are asked to rate 50 child-related situations as problematic or nonproblematic and then to indicate the magnitude of anger elicited in each scenario, using a 5-point scale. This measure has been recommended in identifying anger-control problems and for evaluating treatment effects for anger-reduction intervention. DeRoma and Hansen suggest a possible clinical cutoff score of 148 on the scale measuring magnitude of anger. The Eyberg Child Behavior Inventory (ECBI; Eyberg & Ross, 1978; Eyberg & Colvin, 1994) is a widely used rating scale that measures disruptive behaviors in children aged 2 to 16 and that can be used repeatedly to assess change in behavior over time. Thirty-six common child behavior problems are rated on a 7-point scale for intensity. Parents are then asked to rate whether each behavior is a problem, providing a frequency score. Cutoff scores of 11 on the problem scale and 127 on the intensity scale are suggested. The ECBI has been shown to be sensitive to treatment effects. It should be stated that this measure is limited to conduct-disorder-related behaviors, such as aggression or impulsivity, and is not sensitive to internalizing problems, such as anxiety or depression. The Conners' Rating Scales (Conners, 1990), used to assess patterns of problem behavior in children, includes scales for Conduct Disorder, Anxious–Shy, Restless–Disorganized, Learning Problem, Psychosomatic, Obsessive–Compulsive, Antisocial, and Hyperactive–Immature. For the 48-item version used in Project SafeCare, norms are available for children aged 3 to 17. It also includes a 10-item Hyperactivity Index, which measures the extent to which the child displays behaviors indicative of attention-deficit/hyperactivity disorder.

Cultural and language barriers may occur when using some of these measures. Language barriers may limit the use of some of these instruments with some individuals who are served by agencies providing treatment for child abuse and neglect. Although Spanish-language versions of some of these indirect measures are available, research evaluating the validity of the measures with this population is limited. In Project SafeCare, direct measures were translated for use with the large Spanish-speaking population of families in southern California. All materials provided to parents were also made available in Spanish. Evaluations of the three Project SafeCare components further validated their use with Spanish-speaking families (Cordon et al., 1998) Indirect measures for which there was no existing translation were also translated into Spanish by native Spanish speakers. Each translation was double-checked for accuracy by another Spanish speaker, but despite these translations, cultural barriers existed that made some of these measures inappropriate for some families. Several questions were perceived as rude and intrusive by some parents. Some translations did not reflect the true nature of the question. This problem was further complicated because of the various dialects spoken by many of the Spanish-speaking families served by Project SafeCare.

Organizing and Conducting Assessment and Training Sessions

With the components of assessment and treatment outlined, we now discuss methods for organizing these components into a plan. In Project SafeCare, a standard time line of assessment and training components was followed. Generally, health training was conducted first, followed by home safety and cleanliness, and then by PAT. Note that this is not the sequence in which the chapters present these components. We have placed PAT first as a reflection of its importance and relevance to service providers, not as our recommended delivery sequence.

An overview of the content of each of these training components and their related assessments is provided in Table 3.1. We recommend that parent services follow the sequence of health, home safety, and PAT unless there are specific reasons to conduct sessions in a different order. Assessment and training sessions are organized into a series of approximately 19 weekly sessions, or visits. Each session lasts approximately 1 to 2 hours. This series of sessions can be found in Table 3.3. Training components are conducted in this standard order unless there is a specific need to address a problem within a home. In our experience, families accept and value training in infant and child health care for its immediate benefits, and so it should be offered first. On a practical level, the health assessments can be conducted relatively quickly. Further, we have found that this allows a greater amount of time in which counselors and families can build rapport and cooperation before beginning assessments for

TABLE 3.3. General Order of Assessment and Training Sessions

- *Session 1*
- Introduce project staff, give project overview, and get to know each other
- Review and sign consent forms
- Begin completing demographic questionnaire
- Conduct two health role-play scenarios (assessments) and true–false quizzes

Session 2
- Administer Child Abuse Potential Inventory and Parenting Stress Index
- Conduct one health role-play scenario and true–false quiz
- Present health manual to parent and ask parent to read first section

Session 3
- Administer Beck Depression Inventory
- Conduct one health role-play scenario and true–false quiz (if necessary)
- Health Training Session 1

Session 4
- Administer Eyberg Child Behavior Inventory and Parental Anger Inventory (depending on child's age)
- Health Training Session 2

Session 5
- Administer Parent Behavior Checklist and Conners' Rating Scales (depending on child's age)
- Health Training Session 3

Session 6
- Health Training Session 4
- Complete Home Safety and Cleanliness Assessment Participant Consent with parent
- Home Safety/Cleanliness assessment of home

Session 7
- Health Training Session 5
- Ask parent to fill out Health Consumer Satisfaction Questionnaire
- Home Safety/Cleanliness assessment of home

Session 8
- Home Safety/Cleanliness Training session 1 (training session begins with assessment of home)
- Administer Daily Activities Checklist
- Planned Activities and Parent–Child Interaction assessment during play activity

Session 9
- Home Safety/Cleanliness Training session 2 (training session includes assessment of home)
- Planned Activities and Parent–Child Interaction assessment during play activity

Session 10
- Home Safety/Cleanliness Training session 3 (training session includes assessment of home)
- Planned Activities and Parent–Child Interaction assessment during daily routine (meal, bath, or dress)

Session 11
- Home Safety/Cleanliness Training session 4 (training session includes assessment of home)
- Planned Activities and Parent–Child Interaction assessment during daily routine (meal, bath, or dress)

(continued)

TABLE 3.3. (continued)

Session 12
- Home Safety/Cleanliness Training session 5
- Ask parent to fill out Home Safety/Cleanliness Training Consumer Satisfaction Questionnaire
- Planned Activities and Parent–Child Interaction assessment during daily routine (meal, bath, or dress)

Session 13
- Home Safety/Cleanliness post-training assessment of home
- Planned Activities and Parent–Child Interaction Training session 1 (training session begins with an observational assessment of parent–child interactions)

Session 14
- Planned Activities and Parent–Child Interaction Training session 2 (training session begins with an observational assessment of parent–child interactions)

Session 15
- Planned Activities and Parent–Child Interaction Training session 3 (training session begins with an observational assessment of parent–child interactions)

Session 16
- Planned Activities and Parent–Child Interaction Training session 4 (training session begins with an observational assessment of parent–child interactions)

Session 17
- Planned Activities and Parent–Child Interaction Training session 5
- Ask parent to fill out Planned Activities and Parent–Child Interaction Training Consumer Satisfaction Questionnaire
- Administer Child Abuse Potential Inventory and Parenting Stress Index

Session 18
- Post-training assessment of Planned Activities and Parent–Child Interaction (play and one of the following situations: meal, bath, or dress)
- Administer Beck Depression Inventory, Eyberg Child Behavior Inventory, and Parental Anger Inventory

Session 19
- Post-training assessment of Planned Activities and Parent–Child Interaction (observe two of the following situations not observed during previous session: meal, bath, or dress)
- Administer Parent Behavior Checklist (Fox, 1994) and Conners' Rating Scale
- Brief review of three training components
- Presentation of Certificate of Completion and grocery gift certificate

the home safety and planned activities–parent training components. Assessment for these latter components involves looking throughout the home for hazards and observing the parents and children engaging in common activities. These observations are more invasive and involve subject matter that can be considered more sensitive or private than the assessments required of the health component, which can begin on the second visit to the families' homes.

An urgent need to address a specific problem may be one reason for conducting training components in a different order. For example, if a home contains an extreme number of imminently dangerous hazards or is dangerously cluttered, home safety would be the first component addressed. Home safety assessments would be done early in the program, so that home safety training could be conducted before health training. One family was referred to Project SafeCare because their young child had ingested a poisonous substance that was left in an unlocked cabinet under the kitchen sink. The ingestion of this substance caused severe and ongoing medical complications for the child. In this case, home safety and child health care skills were addressed before parent–child interaction skills training began. Thus there is flexibility in this schedule. We recommend that only one training component be conducted at a time. For instance, conducting home safety and health care skills training at the same time may be overwhelming and would most likely be too time-consuming for most families.

Table 3.3 lists the tasks that are completed during each session and the general order in which sessions are conducted. If it is not possible to complete all of the tasks in a given session, they can be carried into the next session. In fact, it was necessary to deviate from this schedule with most of the families in Project SafeCare. Often, the length of time it may take to complete a given assessment or training with one family is different from what it may be for another family for a number of reasons. Families may prefer shorter or longer visits and may require more or less guidance in completing training. It is important, however, to fully involve parents in determining the pace at which these tasks are conducted so that they are aware of the time and response requirement for participation in the project.

In Project SafeCare, the goal for every family was to successfully complete each of the three training components in five training sessions per component. The training protocols are divided into five sessions, but it is certainly possible to revise this schedule to spread out training over several more sessions. Families with working parents did not always have enough time to complete everything in a given session, so tasks were carried over into subsequent sessions, and additional sessions were added at the end to ensure that all training sessions were completed. On the other hand, in some cases, fewer sessions may be conducted. For example, if a home contains only a few hazards or is very clean, home safety training sessions may be condensed so that training addresses two rooms per session instead of one room per session.

It is most important to work with the parents to determine how much can be accomplished in one weekly session, whether it is possible or desirable to meet twice per week, and the number of sessions that are likely to be needed to complete all three training components and related assessment. If parents are not involved in this process or are unaware of the progress they have made and of how much is still required of them, it may be less likely that families continue to participate in services. Asking for feedback from parents on a regular basis, such as at the beginning or end of each meeting, is one way to promote communication about the process of conducting these interventions. In Project SafeCare, a time was set aside at the end of each session for parents to give feedback on whether they felt they had successfully completed the activities of that session and whether the counselors were courteous, helpful, treated the family fairly, and provided clear explanations of what was expected during that session.

In addition to giving parents every opportunity to provide feedback at the end of each session, counselors followed a set of steps in conducting every session with families. These steps are listed on the Family Session Summary (see Chapter 4, Appendix 4.1). On this form, counselors listed the tasks that were to be conducted in a given session. In addition to this agenda, steps that formed a framework for each session were listed. These steps included:

(1) checking to see if a good day to conduct a training session; (2) reviewing previous sessions; (3) stating the purpose of the day's session; (4) identifying the activities for the day; (5) identifying expectations for the parents and the children, as well as the counselor; and, at the end of the session, (6) reviewing the session; (7) providing positive feedback to parents and children; and (8) scheduling the following session.

During the initial greeting and "catching up" time after the counselor arrives at the home, he or she inquires about whether it is a "good day" to conduct a training session. If it appears that family members are ill or are burdened with other, more pressing issues, training may not be conducted that day. Instead, the counselor can suggest that they reschedule for another day and then leave. Alternatively, the counselor may stay and offer assistance in dealing with a particular issue. For example, one family was experiencing a great deal of difficulty due to a serious cockroach and insect infestation in their apartment. They did not know who to talk to in order to help eradicate the problem. Because this issue was clearly preoccupying the family's attention on this day, the counselor suggested not conducting assessment or training on this day and instead offered her assistance in contacting the family's landlord and, if necessary, the health department. The activities previously scheduled for this day were rescheduled for later in the week, and the family was able to promptly deal with this distressing problem, which, if not acknowledged and addressed, may have prevented the family from fully attending to and participating in the training session.

At the beginning of each training session, the counselor gives a brief review of the previous session and tells the family what is scheduled for the current session. The specific activities are described, as well as what may be asked of the parents and the children. The counselor also explains what his or her role will be in that session. Following the session the counselor reviews the current session, and provides specific positive feedback to the children and the parents. For example, an improvement in a parent's use of positive interaction skills with his or her children would be acknowledged, or an instance of cooperation and play between siblings would be pointed out.

In addition to this general framework for conducting a visit with a family, a general format for conducting training with families is set forth. This protocol applies to each of the three training components and provides the counselors with a structure for the training portion of each session. The steps of this framework can be found in Table 3.4. Training within a given session may be broken down into smaller portions in which specific information or skills are taught to parents. Skills or new information are first explained to parents. A rationale is provided for new skills. Then the counselor models the skills for the parent, and the

---

TABLE 3.4. General Training Format

1. Describe desired target behavior or skills.
2. Explain rationale for each behavior.
3. Model each behavior. You may provide further discussion during modeling.
4. Ask parent to practice behavior; observe with checklist.
5. Provide positive feedback. Point out any positive aspect of parent's performance.
6. Provide constructive feedback. Point out aspects of performance needing improvement.
7. Review parent's performance and set goals for the coming week.

parent practices those skills. The counselor provides positive feedback to parents for correct performance of the target skills and then provides constructive feedback and suggestions for improvement when necessary. Positive feedback is always provided, regardless of how close the parent's performance is to criterion. Then, if additional practice is needed, parents are asked to continue practicing, with additional discussion and modeling provided for the parent as needed until the parent demonstrates the target skills correctly. During practice, the counselor uses the appropriate checklist to record the steps that were completed correctly or that need improvement. For example, during health training, the counselor uses the Parent Behavior Checklist (see Appendix 7.7) to check off steps completed correctly by the parent. Then, at the end of each training session, the counselor and the parent review the day's session and set goals for the coming week.

This framework applies each time a new skill is introduced and may actually be put into practice several times within a given session. For example, during PAT, the counselor may explain each step of the PAT checklist individually (i.e., the activity, the rules, the consequences, etc.), describe the rationale for each step, model these steps individually, ask the parent to practice each step, and then offer feedback for each step before moving on to the next step. As described in the training protocol, however, there is flexibility in how much new information and how many new behaviors may be introduced at one time.

Chapters 4 and 5 detail assessment and training protocols for PAT and PCI training. Chapter 6 describes home safety and cleanliness training, and Chapter 7 covers infant and child health care skills. Remember, in the field, the sequence of presentation is usually reversed.

4

Parenting Assessment for Bonding Skills

RATIONALE FOR PARENT TRAINING

Planned Activities Training (PAT) is used to increase positive interactions between parents and children. It was adapted from procedures described by Sanders and Dadds (1982). Originally taught to parents to promote generalization of child management training, PAT was adapted for use as the primary intervention for parents of children with developmental disabilities who demonstrate challenging behaviors (Huynen et al., 1996). In Project SafeCare, PAT was an effective intervention with parents reported for child maltreatment. The basic rationale for PAT is that prevention is better than a cure. Parents are taught to promote appropriate and positive interactions with their children and to prevent challenging child behaviors. This training component involves teaching parents skills they can use to structure activities and increase bonding and attachment within the relationship. The parent learns to plan stimulating play and daily living activities in advance, to prepare the child for these activities, and to engage the child in these activities using effective interaction skills and incidental teaching. By doing so, the parent can prevent challenging child behaviors, and the parent and child are able to enjoy increasingly positive interactions and activities. Assessment related to PAT will be described here. The PAT protocol is described in Chapter 5.

MATERIALS

The following materials are used during assessment and training in the Parent–Child Interactions (PCI)/PAT component. These materials are also used during training, which is described in Chapter 5.

- *Family Session Summary.* As described in Chapter 3, this form lists tasks planned for each session. See Appendix 4.1.
- *Daily Activities Checklist.* This checklist is used to assess the level of difficulty par-

ents experience with their child's behavior in common daily activities. See Appendix 4.2.

- *PAT Checklists*. These checklists are used to assess parents' use of PAT and to provide parents with written prompts of the steps of PAT for a number of activities. Examples are provided here, but they can be modified as needed. See Appendices 4.3 to 4.7.
- *PCI data sheet*. Use this interval data sheet (see Appendix 4.8) when using the more involved time-sampling observation method of assessing the quality of parent–child interactions. (This method is described more fully in a later section.)
- *Interaction Skills Checklist*. Although not used in Project SafeCare, and thus not evaluated for its equivalence to the time-sampling method, this checklist provides a simpler method for evaluating interaction skills. See Appendix 4.9.
- *Activity Cards*. In Project SafeCare, parents were provided with a set of activity cards that provided age-appropriate suggestions for activities in which parents and children can engage and interact. Sample activities are provided in Appendix 4.10. Additional activity cards are available from the authors.
- *PAT Checklist: Encouraging Independent Play When You Are Necessarily Busy*. This PAT checklist outlines the steps parents should take to engage their child in independent activities when parents are busy. See Appendix 4.11.
- *PCI Training Consumer Satisfaction Questionnaire*. This form provides parents the opportunity to give feedback to the counselor on the training procedures and results. See Appendix 4.12.
- *Audiotape player with headphones and audiotapes for use with Interval Recording Procedures*. Counselors listen to these audiotapes with headphones to hear each 10-second observe, 5-second record interval used during the time-sampling observational method counted off. When two counselors are observing at the same time, use a splitter on the tape player so that both observers may listen to the same audiotape. See Appendix 4.13.

PARENTING ASSESSMENT

Before beginning PAT, we conduct an assessment to determine areas in which parents need assistance. Although this is a very structured, well-validated assessment, we still ask the parents about child behaviors that are of concern to them. We do this because parents are usually good judges of the challenging behavior of their children.

Occasionally, a parent's request for a behavior change might be inappropriate because the child is not yet developmentally ready to meet the parent's expectation. For example, some parents in Illinois believed that it was appropriate for a 3-year-old child to sit quietly through a 3- or 4-hour church revival meeting. In cases such as this, the counselor must provide some child development information to the parent and must refuse to create a behavior management program aimed at something for which the child is not developmentally ready.

The assessment sessions involve gathering information about the child's and the parents' behaviors. The Daily Activities Checklist provides a format for gaining the parents' perspective on which situations pose the most challenges in terms of child behavior (see Appendix 4.2). This checklist can guide the counselor and parent in determining in which settings assessment and training should take place. Two of these situations are targeted for training, and at least one other is targeted for generalization observations. Parents are then asked to demonstrate with their child how they interact during the identified challenging situations, such as playtime or mealtime. By observing parents and children interacting during such activities, the counselor is more effectively able to assess the quality of the interactions, how parents engage their children in activities, and their children's responses.

There are two parts to these assessment observations: the interaction skills assessment and the PAT assessment. The interaction skills assessment, which evaluates parents' and children's use of appropriate verbalizations, touches, and other skills, can be somewhat time-consuming and labor intensive. The reason is that the research protocol used in Project SafeCare calls for procedures that yield very detailed information. These procedures, however, can be modified to suit individual needs. We discuss such modifications later. The PAT assessment involves the use of 10-item checklists (see Appendices 4.3–4.7). This type of assessment is much easier and simpler to do, although it does not necessarily capture the skills that are addressed by the interaction skills observational procedures. A simplified way of conducting the interaction skills assessment is discussed later in this chapter.

During the assessment, at least four to five baseline observations are conducted. These observations are done across different situations, such as playtime, bath time, mealtime, and getting dressed. Observations may be conducted during any activity, either in the home or the community, but the PAT checklist may need to be modified for different activities. *Note: The steps on each of the activity checklists are essentially the same, with the exception of the examples and suggestions listed under each heading.*

GUIDELINES FOR CONDUCTING OBSERVATIONS

The selection of observation settings and of the settings in which training is conducted should be guided by the parent's report of which settings are most problematic. This can be determined by having the parent complete the Daily Activities Checklist. In Project SafeCare, observations were conducted in the families' homes, but they may be conducted in any number of home and community settings, such as the grocery store, physician's or dentist's office, or while riding in the car. Observations should be conducted for a minimum of 10 minutes; however, if the activity requires more time, such as mealtime or bath time, the observation should continue until the activity is over. All observations should include the behaviors that the parent engages in to begin and to end an activity so that the counselor can assess the skills that make up PAT.

Materials

To conduct a baseline observation, you will need the following materials:

- PCI data sheet (interval data sheet if using time sampling method; skills checklist if using simpler method).
- PAT checklists (preprepared checklists or your own).

- Audiocassette player and earphones and 10-second observe, 5-second-record cassette tape (if using the time sampling method; see Appendix 4.13) (optional).
- Pencil.
- Clipboard.
- Toys (age appropriate, for play situations; bring from office if necessary).

Provide Rationale to the Parent

Before conducting the baseline observations, provide the parent with a rationale for the observations. The rationale should include the following point:

"In order to conduct a thorough service, we ask you to show us how you interact with your child, and how your child behaves in a variety of situations."

Preparing for the Observation

The steps for conducting an observation follow.

- *Instructions to the parent.* Give the following instruction to the parent before beginning the observation:

"We would like to watch while you and your child _____ [name the activity, e.g., play, eat lunch, prepare for nap time]. We will watch for at least 10 minutes, or until you are finished. During that time, we want you to do whatever you would normally do to begin and end the activity, as well as what you normally do during the activity. We want you to interact with your child as you normally would. Please try to pretend that I am not here. Unless you need to talk to us about something important, please wait until the observation is over."

- *Instructions to the child.* If the child is old enough to understand, give age-appropriate instructions to child about what will happen and what is expected of him or her. For example, tell the child that it is time for her or him to play with her or his mother and that you want her or him to pretend that you are not there. Do not provide the child with any additional prompts or incentives, such as how he or she should behave or what will happen after the observation.
- Ask the parent to begin.
- If the parent talks to you during the observation about something that is not urgent, ask her or him to wait until the observation is over. If the child approaches you or other staff members during the observation, direct him or her back to the parent.
- At the end of the observation, thank the parent and the child for participating.

Note: It is important to capture the behaviors the parent and child engage in during transition times, as well as during activities. That is, you want to observe what happens when they begin an activity, end an activity, or move from one activity to the next. Therefore, always begin the observation as the parent and child begin the activity and continue observing until the parent and child have completed the activity and are about to begin the next activity, even if the observation lasts longer than 10 minutes. If a parent ends an activity abruptly, ask her or him if that is always how the activity ends. If she or he says "Yes," end the observation. If she or he says "No" and indicates that she or he would do something different, ask her or him to show how the activity would normally end. Note on the data sheet that the observation was interrupted and that the counselor provided a prompt to end the activity. Record until parent indicates that she or he has completed what she or he normally does.

USING THE PAT CHECKLISTS

The PAT checklists assess the parents' use of PAT in specific daily living activities. The counselor should complete the checklist when observing parent–child activities. The parent should demonstrate each step of the checklist according to the definitions in the next session. Place a "+" in the box if the parent completes the step correctly. Place a "−" in the box if the parent completes the steps incorrectly or does not complete the step at all. If a particular step is not applicable to an activity, write in "N/A." Then calculate a percentage score. Divide the number of steps completed correctly ("+") by the total number of steps. Then multiply by 100 to get a "percent correct" score.

Planned Activities Definitions

The following are general operational definitions for each step on the PAT checklists. The checklists are used to assess parent performance of PAT and to provide a written prompt to parents about steps to take while interacting with their child. For each activity checklist presented to parents, each step should be tailored to the family's specific needs. For example, specific rules and reinforcers should be selected and listed under the appropriate step on the checklist to make each list useful for parents engaging in specific activities.

Prepare in Advance

The parent takes steps to have an activity prepared in advance. This may involve planning to involve the child in preparations, making preparations that the child will not be involved in before beginning the activity, giving advance warning of an activity, or having necessary supplies ready prior to beginning an activity.
Examples:

- Setting towels and clothes out before bath time.
- Planning to have the child help put napkins on the table while the parent sets the table.
- Giving advance warning to the child that lunch will be ready soon.

Explain Activity

The parent explains, describes, or names an activity prior to or at the beginning of the activity.

Examples:

- "After we pick up these toys we are going to have a snack."
- "Let's play with your train now."
- "Jamie, first we are going to brush our teeth and then we will read a story."
- "We're going to get dressed now."

Explain the Rules

The parent explains what is expected of the child in a given activity; that is, the behaviors in which the child should and should not engage. Rules should be stated positively, indicating what the child should do rather than not do (e.g., "Keep your feet on the floor" rather than "Don't put your feet on the table"). *Note: In order for the behavior to be scored on the PAT checklist as occurring appropriately, the parent must provide positive rules.*

Examples:

- "Touch nicely while we play house. Now what do we need to do?"
- "Crayons are for drawing on paper only. Where are we going to draw?"
- "Toys should be picked up when you are finished"
- "Keep your hands to yourself and stay with me while we are in the store."
- "Finish all of your cereal."

Explain the Consequences

The parent calmly explains the consequences for following and not following the rules before beginning a given activity.

Examples:

- "If you keep your hands to yourself, you can play with the puzzle."
- "When you pick up the toys, we can go outside and play."
- "If you throw the blocks, we have to put them away."
- "If you don't sit on your bottom in the chair, you might fall down."

Give Choices

The parent provides a choice within the activity.

Examples:

- Choice of food items ("Do you want one or two scoops of rice?")
- Choice of clothing items ("Do you want the blue or the red shirt?")

- Choice of times ("Do you want to eat now or later?")
- Choice of who will help the child ("Do you want your dad or me to help?")

Talk about What You Are Doing (Incidental Teaching)

The parent takes advantage of natural, unplanned opportunities to engage the child in the activity by using language. The interaction should be directed by the child and should be brief, positive, and focused on the child-selected activity or items. It should also involve language that is age appropriate for the child.

Examples:

- While the child is coloring, the parent describes the colors the child is using or the content of the picture.
- While the child is playing with dolls, the parent asks questions about what the dolls are doing.
- While eating breakfast, the parent talks about healthy foods the child enjoys.
- While the child is getting dressed, the parent asks the child about the colors of his or her clothing.
- While driving in the car, the parent gives brief and simple explanations about the trucks the child sees on the road.

Use Good Interaction Skills

The parent levels (gets eye-to-eye with child) and uses appropriate verbalizations, facial expression, and touch. (With the PAT checklists, these behaviors are assessed in a more general fashion. See specific definitions in the section on interaction skills assessment.)

Ignore Minor Misbehavior

The parent ignores minor inappropriate behavior in which the child engages. Minor misbehavior refers to behaviors that do not result in the child or another individual being hurt or items being broken. By "ignore," we mean that the parent should not attend to the inappropriate behavior in which the child is engaged but should withdraw his or her attention for a brief period, as if he or she is attending to other matters. During this time, however, the parent should not ignore behavior that will result in harm to the child or other individuals. In these situations, the child should be redirected to more appropriate behaviors.

Give Feedback

Feedback refers to descriptive statements made by the parent and directed to the child regarding the child's performance. It refers to an evaluation of the child's behavior or attributes or to an activity, behavior, or product of the child. Feedback should be clear and descriptive. Feedback should also be positive, but when describing inappropriate behavior, it should provide a description of the behavior that the child should demonstrate in that situation.

Examples:

- "You placed the towel on the counter. Great job."
- "You kept your food on your plate."
- "You did not keep your hands to yourself when we were in the store. Next time remember to keep your hands to yourself."

Provide Rewards or Consequences

Rewards or consequences refer to reinforcing items or activities provided to the child during or immediately following an activity. This may involve tangible items, such as toys or snacks, or opportunities to engage in desired activities that are provided contingent on appropriate child behavior. Appropriate use of consequences may also involve withholding reinforcers when appropriate. Remember that for younger children, rewards should be immediate rather than delayed.

USING THE PARENT–CHILD INTERACTION SKILLS DATA SHEETS

This section describes the procedures used to assess parent–child interaction skills in Project SafeCare. *For research purposes, some of the assessment procedures were very detailed and demanding and required a great deal of training time. For this reason, they may not be appropriate for purely clinical or teaching purposes. These procedures are described here, and suggestions for modifying these procedures to make them more user-friendly follow the descriptions.*

These skills can be assessed using a time-sampling method, described later, or may be fashioned into a general checklist. The definitions are provided because they have been validated by professionals as being important to assess when evaluating the quality of parent–child interaction skills.

Recording Intervals

The PCI data sheet is arranged for recording the occurrence of parent and child behaviors in 10-second intervals. See Appendix 4.8 for a copy of the data sheet used in Project SafeCare. The data sheets are designed to be used with a 10-second-observe, 5-second-record partial interval recording system. This means that observers watch the parent and child interact for 10 seconds, looking for all of the target behaviors, and then record for 5 seconds. The observer does not write anything down on the data sheet during the observation interval. He or she only watches the interaction. Then, when the 5-second record interval begins, the observer looks down and checks off each of the behaviors he or she observed. This requires remembering each behavior during that 10-second interval. After recording for 5 seconds, he or she observes again for 10 seconds and then records for 5 seconds. To cue the observer when to observe and record, he or she listens to a prerecorded audiotape with headphones. A tape designed to be used during a 10-minute observation should include cues for 40 intervals (4 observe–record intervals per minute). This tape counts off the beginning of each 10-second-observe interval and each 5-second-record interval. See Appendix 4.13 for instructions on making such an audiotape.

Recording Procedures

The prerecorded cassette tape, played on a small tape player with headphones, cues the observer to observe and record at the correct times. The interval number and condition are stated. That is, the tape starts with "Observe 1" to indicate that the observer is to watch and that this is the first interval. This is followed by "Record 1," indicating that the observer should now record the behaviors just observed in the space for Interval 1 on the data sheet. Each interval is marked in this manner up to interval 40. If the observation continues beyond 40 intervals (i.e., beyond 10 minutes), the observer will need to restart the tape and begin a new data sheet. During the observation, the observer should sit at a distance that is not intrusive in the parent's and child's interactions but is close enough to the dyad to hear the parent and child and to be able to see facial expressions and other behaviors. The observer should not become involved in the parent–child interaction but should remain as unobtrusive as possible. If children approach the observer during the observation, the observer should explain that he or she has writing to do and direct the child back to the activity.

If a behavior occurs at all, for any length of time, within a 10-second interval, it is recorded in the corresponding space on the data sheet. The behavior *does not* have to occur throughout the entire interval to be scored as occurring. The behavior *does* have to occur during the "observe" interval. If a behavior happens to occur only during a record interval, its occurrence should not be recorded.

Behaviors should be scored in the following manner. Occurrence of a behavior is indicated by making a slash (in pencil) through the corresponding letter or by making a slash through the "+" or "−" signs (as defined later). When the "+" or "−" sign is marked, the letter code is not marked. Nonoccurrence of a behavior is indicated by *not* marking the corresponding code.

Data Sheet

To use the data sheet, complete the information at the top of the form:

- *Parent and Child.* Record the names of those involved in the interaction.
- *Setting/Activity.* Record the place where the observation is being conducted and the activity in which the parent and child are engaged—for example, eating breakfast in the kitchen, playing in the backyard, shopping at the grocery store, or walking at the park.
- *Observer.* Record the name of the observer
- *(P R).* Indicate whether the observer is the primary data collector (P) or an additional observer (R) collecting data concurrently with the primary observer in order to assess interobserver reliability.
- *Condition.* Indicate the experimental condition the observation was conducted in by circling Bl—baseline, Trtmt—training, or Follow-up

Simplified Strategies for Assessing Interaction Skills

A more simplified, yet less precise, method for evaluating parent and child interaction skills is to formulate a checklist that includes each of the interaction skills in the following list. During an observation of parent–child interactions, the counselor should check off each skill that was demonstrated correctly. A sample of this checklist can be found in Appendix 4.9. This checklist may be used in an informal fashion to make notes about specific skills parents demonstrate or may need to practice. It may also be used to count the number of times parents demonstrate each of these skills in a given time period. This checklist has not been empirically validated as a measure of interaction skills, and therefore there are no specific rules regarding how data collected using this checklist should be interpreted. Rather than a formal assessment measure, it can be used as a tool to structure observations that may otherwise be unstructured.

Definitions of Parent Interaction Skills

L: Leveling

Parent assumes a physical position that approximates the height of the child so that he or she is able to make horizontal eye contact. The parent's eyes should be no more that one foot above or below those of the child.

Examples:

- Parent kneels next to child.
- Parent sits on the floor.
- Parent sits next to the child on the couch.
- Parent has child on his or her lap.
- Parent holds the child.

AT: Attending

Parent is directing his or her attention toward the child and his or her activity. This also involves being within approximately 3 to 4 feet of the child, unless the specific activity precludes this, such as hide-and-go-seek or jump rope. The parent should be engaged in activity or conversation that directly involves the child in order for attending to be scored.

T: Touch

+T: APPROPRIATE TOUCH

Any direct physical contact between persons (or their clothing) in an affectionate, gentle, pleasant, or helping manner.

Examples: Hugging, cuddling, kissing, patting, stroking, tickling, gentle bouncing, sitting on parent's lap, holding hands, sitting next to a child, or having arms around the child.

–T: INAPPROPRIATE TOUCH

Any direct physical contact made by the adult to the children that is rough, painful, constraining, or restraining.

Examples: Hitting, spanking, jerking, pulling, and grabbing tightly, attempting to hug the child when the child is struggling to move away from the parent.

Note: Touch is scored for the parent when initiated by either the parent or the child. If touch is initiated by the child and the parent has accepted the touch or reciprocated, this is also scored as a touch for the parent.

V: Verbal

+V: APPROPRIATE VERBAL

Verbal statements made in a respectful tone and directed toward the child; includes discussion, questions, answers to questions, descriptions, interpretations, elaborations, stories, attention statements, instructions, commands, praise, or requests. In order for the behavior to be scored as appropriate, the parent must demonstrate congruence between his or her affect and verbal statement.

Examples:

- "What are you going to do with the doll?" [asked in a curious tone]
- "Oh, look, you're stacking the blocks."
- "Hi, sweetheart."
- "You're doing great!"
- "Now it's time to brush your teeth."
- "Keep your hands to yourself."

–V: INAPPROPRIATE VERBAL

Any verbal comments or vocal noises that are negative in content or tone directed toward the children by the adult. This includes complaining, yelling, screaming, arguing, whining, crying, repeatedly questioning the child when the child has already answered or will not answer, calling the child's name without saying anything further, threatening, or calling the children a derogatory or disrespectful name.

Examples:

- "Shut up."
- "Sue, Sue, Sue . . . "
- "Cut it out."
- "Why do you always do that?"

In: Instructions

+IN: APPROPRIATE INSTRUCTIONS

Any verbal utterance emitted by the adult that sets the occasion for the child to immediately terminate an extreme form of a given behavior or to immediately engage in a more acceptable form of a given behavior. Instructions should be stated clearly and positively, with appropriate voice quality (firm, but not mean), and should be simple (2–10 simple words within child's vocabulary) and specific. Parents should give the child an opportunity to respond following the instruction and refer to one response at a time.

This does not include suggestions that are within the context of a play situation, such as "draw a green circle."

Examples:

- "Put your toys away."
- "It is time to go to bed."

–IN: INAPPROPRIATE INSTRUCTIONS

Instructions that are nonspecific, do not give the child an opportunity to follow the instruction, are stated negatively, consist of gestures only, are overly complex (11+ words), or are inappropriate for the child's vocabulary.

Examples:

- Parent uses only gestures or facial expression to communicate with the child.
- "If you don't stop, I am going to send you to your room. You know you aren't supposed to do that."
- "Pick these up . . . pick these up . . . " (without giving child an opportunity to respond before a second instruction).

Note: Instructions should include each aspect of the definition in order to be scored as appropriate. An instruction in which the content is appropriate but that is given in an inappropriately angry or mean tone is scored as inappropriate. In this case, a negative verbal is also scored.

IT: Incidental Teaching

Incidental teaching takes advantage of natural, unplanned opportunities to engage the child in a variety of activities and to increase the use of language. The interaction should be directed by the child and should be brief, positive, and focused on the child-selected activity or items. It should also involve language that is age appropriate for the child. Incidental teaching can involve elaborating on the activity in which the child is engaged, encouraging the child to use his or her language, suggesting ways of expanding on the activity in which the child is engaged, asking questions about the activity in which the child is engaged or showing interest, or describing the activity in which the child is engaged. The parent should not be overly concerned with directing the activity or trying to "teach" the child something new. The parent should not insist on the child following the suggestion but should use the suggestion to facilitate the child's exploration.

Examples:

- "Where do you put your arms?" (while the child is putting on a shirt)
- "What do we do next?" (after the child puts toothpaste on the toothbrush)
- "What should we do with these cups?"
- "Look, you put the soap on your feet." (while the child is taking a bath)
- "What color are these apples?" (while grocery shopping)
- "We can build a house with the blocks."
- "Let's soak up the water with the sponge."
- "What kind of animal is that?"
- "You're right, that's a dog."
- "Why don't we stack the cups and make a tower?"
- "Let's add the flour to the cookie dough and see what happens"

Definitions of Child Interaction Skills

V: Verbal

+V: APPROPRIATE VERBAL

A question, answer, interpretation, elaboration, story, attention statement, or vocal noise. These include requests for information regarding any of the days activities, planned activities or routines, and remarks about school, work, or social occasions.

Examples:

- "When is lunch?" (questioning)
- "Can we go outside?"
- "We went to the park."
- "The house is tall."
- "I want some juice."

−V: INAPPROPRIATE VERBAL

Any defiant, socially unacceptable, or disrespectful statements, comments, or vocal noises made by the children.

Examples:

- Refusals to do something, complaining, whining, demanding, yelling, screaming, arguing, crying, repeatedly questioning something that the adult has already denied, repeatedly calling the adult's name (twice within 3 seconds or once without saying anything further, e.g., "Mom, Mom, . . . "), threatening, warning, calling another person a derogatory or disrespectful name, including foul language.
- "When's lunch?!" (demanding)

- "I don't want to." (whining)
- "Mom, Mom, Mom . . . "
- "I want to go outside!" (yelling, whining, arguing, or repeating)

Note: Verbal statements are scored according to content, not affect. Affect is scored separately.

A: Affect

+A: POSITIVE AFFECT

Modulation in a child's voice which is indicative of positive emotion. A child's facial expression is also useful in identifying positive affect.
   Examples: Smiling, laughing, giggling, talking cheerfully.
   Note: Neutral affect is scored as positive affect.

–A: NEGATIVE AFFECT

Verbalizations or noises in which voice modulation is indicative of negative emotions. A child's facial expression is useful in identifying negative affect.
   Examples: Inappropriate harsh yelling, whining, crying, sarcasm, screaming, pouting, frowning, scowling, glaring.

AG: Physical Aggression

Any physical contact or gesture to make such contact with or toward another person or animal in a manner that could cause harm or discomfort or is likely to if that behavior continues.
   Examples: The child physically strikes, grabs, kicks, pushes, trips, swings, spits at, bites, pulls hair of, pinches, scratches, or throws something at (not to, as in playing catch) another person or animal. Attempts to engage in these behaviors are also scored as aggression.

FI: Following Instructions

After an appropriate instruction by the adult, the child begins the appropriately requested behavior within 30 seconds of the first instruction.
   Note: Following instructions should be scored within the interval in which it occurs, not necessarily the interval in which the instruction occurred. Following instructions should be scored, if it occurs, even when the parent gave the instruction inappropriately.

Additional Notes

For children only, any verbal utterance may be scored in any combination with any affect.
   Examples:

- +V, +A: "Mom, let's have lunch now?" (in a calm, question-like voice)
- +V, –A: "Mom, I want lunch now!!" (in a loud and angry voice)

- −V, +A: "I will not brush my teeth." (while laughing and smiling)
- −V, −A: "You can't make me do that!!" (yelling, after asked to take a bath)

Each of the PAT behaviors, incidental teaching, and imitations is also scored as a *verbal statement*. The category *verbal* is not an exclusive category within the parent and child behavioral categories. Anything the parent says is scored as a verbal. This may include explaining activities, rules, and consequences, providing feedback, or using incidental teaching.

Data Summary

PCI data should be calculated and summarized immediately after each observation. Use the following method to calculate the percentage of intervals in which each behavior occurred:

1. Count intervals occurred. For each behavior, count the number of intervals in which the behavior occurred. Also do this for both positive emitting and negative emitting of the behavior (count the number of intervals in which positive verbal occurred and the number of intervals in which negative verbal occurred).
2. For each category of behavior, divide the number of intervals in which the behavior occurred by the total number of intervals scored. The total number of intervals is the total number of intervals in which observation and recording took place. Intervals that were skipped or not scored should be subtracted from this total.
3. Then multiply the answer by 100 to obtain the percentage score.
4. You then have a percentage score for each behavior within a given observation period. Record these scores on a summary sheet and then graph the data.
5. The data can also be summarized for total appropriate behaviors by adding the numerators and denominators for each appropriate behavior together and then dividing and multiplying by 100. This can be done for all inappropriate behaviors also.

Graphing Data

This step is essential and should be completed after each meeting in which observations take place. The percentage of steps completed correctly on the PAT checklists should be calculated ([number of steps completed correctly/total number of steps possible] × 100) and graphed. This percentage should be placed on a graph labeled "Percentage Correct on PAT Checklist."

The PCI data can be graphed in the same manner by graphing the percent of intervals in which appropriate or inappropriate behavior occurred, the percentage of instructions delivered positively (for parent), and the percentage of instructions followed (for child).

Interobserver Agreement

Interobserver agreement observations should be conducted for at least 25% of the observations. It is important to know that observers are in agreement as to what is being observed and recorded. Interobserver agreement should be calculated immediately following each reliability observation. Calculate agreement data for the data collected during interval recording and use of the PAT checklist by dividing the number of agreements by the number of agreements plus disagreements, then multiply by 100. An agreement is recorded when both observers record that a behavior *has occurred.* That is, only intervals in which either the primary observer or the reliability observer or both have marked a given behavior as occurring are used in determining agreements or disagreements. This will yield a percentage called *occurrence reliability*.

Reliability data are computed for each behavior as follows:

1. Count the number of intervals in which the behavior was recorded as occurring by *both* the primary and reliability observers (Agreements).
2. Count the number of intervals in which the behavior was recorded as occurring by either the primary observer or the reliability observer (Agreements + Disagreements).
3. Divide the number obtained in Step 1 by the number obtained in Step 2 (i.e., Agreements/[Agreements + Disagreements]).
4. Multiply the number obtained in Step 3 by 100 to yield the percentage agreement.
5. Acceptable interobserver agreement percentages are 85% or greater. If agreement percentage is less than that, additional training in the observational procedures should be conducted.

$$\text{Percentage Agreement} = \frac{A}{A + D} \times 100$$

Family Session Summary

Called 30 minutes prior to appointment
☐ OK ☐ Reschedule ☐ No

Family name _____ Date _____

Adults present _____ Time _____

Children present _____ Staff present _____

_____

_____

Tasks family was to complete during past week:	Completed/Not completed

Agenda for this session:	Data collected		Reliability	
1. _____	Y	N	Y	N
2. _____	Y	N	Y	N
3. _____	Y	N	Y	N
4. _____	Y	N	Y	N
5. _____	Y	N	Y	N

Check box if completed:

☐ Check to see if it is a "good day."
☐ Review previous session.
☐ State purpose of today's session.
☐ Identify today's activities.
☐ Describe parent's role in today's activities.
☐ Describe child's role in today's activities.
☐ Describe counselor's role in today's activities.
☐ Review today's session (after completion).
☐ Provide positive feedback to parent.
☐ Provide positive feedback to children.
☐ Schedule next session—date, time, location.

Notes:

Consumer satisfaction: (ask parent to complete this section)

At this visit, do you feel: Comments

You successfully completed the activity?   Yes   No

The staff member . . .

Was courteous?   Yes   No

Was helpful?   Yes   No

Treated you fairly?   Yes   No

Provided clear explanations of what   Yes   No
        was expected during the session?

Parent _____ Counselor _____

Daily Activities Checklist

Parent: _____   Date: ____ / ____ / ____

Child: _____ Age: _____ Interviewer: _____ Condition: Bl Trtmt Follow-up

Instructions: Identify those situations in which you have experienced difficulty with your child's behavior during the past two weeks. Indicate the extent of change you would like to see in your child's behavior or in the situation.

Situation	OK as is		Some change		Great change	Notes
Waking	1	2	3	4	5	
Getting dressed	1	2	3	4	5	
Mealtimes	1	2	3	4	5	
Meal preparation times	1	2	3	4	5	
Using the bathroom	1	2	3	4	5	
Bath time	1	2	3	4	5	
When you are busy with household chores, talking on the phone, etc.	1	2	3	4	5	
Getting ready to go out	1	2	3	4	5	
When you have visitors	1	2	3	4	5	
Playtime	1	2	3	4	5	
Watching TV	1	2	3	4	5	
Getting ready for bed	1	2	3	4	5	
Bedtime	1	2	3	4	5	
Late evening	1	2	3	4	5	
Doctor/dentist appointments	1	2	3	4	5	
Other appointments	1	2	3	4	5	
Shopping/errands	1	2	3	4	5	
Other community outings: (specify) _____	1	2	3	4	5	
Leaving your child	1	2	3	4	5	
Other (specify) _____	1	2	3	4	5	

Adapted from Sanders and Dadds (1993).

Planned Activities Training Checklist: Playtime

Parent: _____   Date ____ / ____ / ____   Time: _____

Child: _____   Observer: _____ (P R)

Setting/Activity: _____   Condition: Bl   Trtmt   Follow-up

+ Completed correctly
– Completed incorrectly or not completed
N/A Not applicable

Prepare in advance
    Get supplies ready in advance
    Have a plan for what you are going to do	

Explain activity Remember to gain your child's attention	
Explain the rules Simple, clear, and easy to follow	

Explain the consequences
    For following rules
    For not following rules	

Give choices Choice of activities, materials, where to play	

Talk about what you are doing
    Ask questions, but follow your child's lead
    Describe what your child is doing	

Use good interaction skills
    On child's level   Touch
    Calm voice Calm facial expression	

Ignore minor misbehavior Remember to pay attention to good behavior	

Give feedback
    Describe what your child did that was great
    What should he or she work on next time?	

Provide rewards/consequences
    Natural rewards
    Praise, activities, and your attention	

Percent correct:	

Planned Activities Training Checklist: Bath Time

Parent: _____   Date ____ / ____ / ____   Time: ____

Child: _____   Observer: _____ (P R)

Setting/Activity: _____   Condition: Bl   Trtmt   Follow-up

+ Completed correctly
– Completed incorrectly or not completed
N/A Not applicable

Prepare in advance 　　　Have supplies in advance 　　　Give advance warning	
Explain activity 　　　Remember to gain your child's attention	
Explain the rules	
Explain the consequences 　　　For following rules 　　　For not following rules	
Give choices 　　　Wash alone or with help 　　　Wash arms or legs first	
Talk about what you are doing 　　　"Where are your fingers, toes, ears, nose?" 　　　Talk about toys	
Use good interaction skills 　　　On child's level　　　Touch 　　　Calm voice　　　Calm facial expression	
Ignore minor misbehavior	
Give feedback 　　　Describe what your child did that was great 　　　What should he or she work on next time?	
Provide rewards/consequences 　　　Natural rewards 　　　Special book, toy, or game	
Percent correct:	

Planned Activities Training Checklist: Bedtime

Parent: _____

Child: _____

Setting/Activity: _____

Date ____ / ____ / ____   Time: ____

Observer: _____ (P R)

Condition: Bl   Trtmt   Follow-up

+ Completed correctly
− Completed incorrectly or not completed
N/A Not applicable

Prepare in advance
    Get pajamas ready in advance
    Tell child in advance that it is almost bedtime	

Explain activity Remember to gain your child's attention	
Explain the rules	

Explain the consequences
    For following rules
    For not following rules	

Give choices Choice in nighttime stuffed animal, pajamas, story	

Talk about what you are doing
    Read a book, look at pictures ,and talk quietly
    Talk about the day	

Use good interaction skills
    On child's level   Touch
    Calm voice Calm facial expression	

Ignore minor misbehavior
    If child gets up, redirecting him or her back to bed with little
        attention	

Give feedback
    Describe what your child did that was great
    What should he or she work on next time?	

Provide rewards/consequences
    Natural rewards
    Stay positive; attend to good behavior	

Percent correct:	

Planned Activities Training Checklist: Getting Dressed

Parent: _____ Date ____ / ____ / ____ Time: ____

Child: _____ Observer: _____ (P R)

Setting/Activity: _____ Condition: Bl   Trtmt   Follow-up

+ Completed correctly
– Completed incorrectly or not completed
N/A Not applicable

Prepare in advance
    Have clothes ready in advance
    Give advance warning	

Explain activity Remember to gain your child's attention	
Explain the rules	

Explain the consequences
    For following rules
    For not following rules	

Give choices Choice of two clothing items	

Talk about what you are doing
    "What are the colors?"
    "Where are your arms, legs, etc.?"	

Use good interaction skills
    On child's level   Touch
    Calm voice Calm facial expression	

Ignore minor misbehavior	

Give feedback
    Describe what your child did that was great
    What should he or she work on next time?	

Provide rewards/consequences
    Natural rewards
    Special book, toy, or game	

Percent correct:	

Planned Activities Training Checklist: Mealtime

Parent: _____   Date ____ / ____ / ____   Time: _____

Child: _____   Observer: _____ (P R)

Setting/Activity: _____   Condition: Bl   Trtmt   Follow-up

\+ Completed correctly
− Completed incorrectly or not completed
N/A Not applicable

Prepare in advance
    Give few snacks/drinks before mealtime
    Have everything ready before sitting down	

Explain activity Remember to gain your child's attention	
Explain the rules	

Explain the consequences
    For following rules
    For not following rules	

Give choices Choice in food or amount	
Talk about what you are doing The food, the day, plans for the evening	

Use good interaction skills
    On child's level   Touch
    Calm voice Calm facial expression	

Ignore minor misbehavior
    If child refuses to eat, give a few instructions to eat, no rewards
      for refusing	

Give feedback
    Describe what your child did that was great
    What should he or she work on next time?	

Provide rewards/consequences
    Natural rewards
    Stay positive; attend to good behavior	

Percent correct:	

Parent–Child Interactions

Parent: _____   Date ____ / ____ / ____

Child: _____   Time Beg: _____

Setting/Activity: _____   Time End: _____

Observer: _____   (P R) Condition: Bl Trtmt Follow-up

+ Appropriate
– Inappropriate

Parent
L   Leveling
AT   Attending
T   Touch
V   Verbal
In   Instructions
IT   Incidental Teaching

Child
V   Verbal
A   Affect
AG   Aggression
FI   Following Instructions

	PARENT						CHILD				NOTES
1	L	AT	+T–	+V–	+In–	IT	+V–	+A–	AG	FI	
2	L	AT	+T–	+V–	+In–	IT	+V–	+A–	AG	FI	
3	L	AT	+T–	+V–	+In–	IT	+V–	+A–	AG	FI	
4	L	AT	+T–	+V–	+In–	IT	+V–	+A–	AG	FI	
5	L	AT	+T–	+V–	+In–	IT	+V–	+A–	AG	FI	
6	L	AT	+T–	+V–	+In–	IT	+V–	+A–	AG	FI	
7	L	AT	+T–	+V–	+In–	IT	+V–	+A–	AG	FI	
8	L	AT	+T–	+V–	+In–	IT	+V–	+A–	AG	FI	
9	L	AT	+T–	+V–	+In–	IT	+V–	+A–	AG	FI	
10	L	AT	+T–	+V–	+In–	IT	+V–	+A–	AG	FI	
11	L	AT	+T–	+V–	+In–	IT	+V–	+A–	AG	FI	
12	L	AT	+T–	+V–	+In–	IT	+V–	+A–	AG	FI	
13	L	AT	+T–	+V–	+In–	IT	+V–	+A–	AG	FI	
14	L	AT	+T–	+V–	+In–	IT	+V–	+A–	AG	FI	
15	L	AT	+T–	+V–	+In–	IT	+V–	+A–	AG	FI	
16	L	AT	+T–	+V–	+In–	IT	+V–	+A–	AG	FI	
17	L	AT	+T–	+V–	+In–	IT	+V–	+A–	AG	FI	
18	L	AT	+T–	+V–	+In–	IT	+V–	+A–	AG	FI	
19	L	AT	+T–	+V–	+In–	IT	+V–	+A–	AG	FI	
20	L	AT	+T–	+V–	+In–	IT	+V–	+A–	AG	FI	
21	L	AT	+T–	+V–	+In–	IT	+V–	+A–	AG	FI	
22	L	AT	+T–	+V–	+In–	IT	+V–	+A–	AG	FI	
23	L	AT	+T–	+V–	+In–	IT	+V–	+A–	AG	FI	
24	L	AT	+T–	+V–	+In–	IT	+V–	+A–	AG	FI	

(continued)

	PARENT						CHILD				NOTES
25	L	AT	+T–	+V–	+In–	IT	+V–	+A–	AG	FI	
26	L	AT	+T–	+V–	+In–	IT	+V–	+A–	AG	FI	
27	L	AT	+T–	+V–	+In–	IT	+V–	+A–	AG	FI	
28	L	AT	+T–	+V–	+In–	IT	+V–	+A–	AG	FI	
29	L	AT	+T–	+V–	+In–	IT	+V–	+A–	AG	FI	
30	L	AT	+T–	+V–	+In–	IT	+V–	+A–	AG	FI	
31	L	AT	+T–	+V–	+In–	IT	+V–	+A–	AG	FI	
32	L	AT	+T–	+V–	+In–	IT	+V–	+A–	AG	FI	
33	L	AT	+T–	+V–	+In–	IT	+V–	+A–	AG	FI	
34	L	AT	+T–	+V–	+In–	IT	+V–	+A–	AG	FI	
35	L	AT	+T–	+V–	+In–	IT	+V–	+A–	AG	FI	
36	L	AT	+T–	+V–	+In–	IT	+V–	+A–	AG	FI	
37	L	AT	+T–	+V–	+In–	IT	+V–	+A–	AG	FI	
38	L	AT	+T–	+V–	+In–	IT	+V–	+A–	AG	FI	
39	L	AT	+T–	+V–	+In–	IT	+V–	+A–	AG	FI	
40	L	AT	+T–	+V–	+In–	IT	+V–	+A–	AG	FI	
Total											
% score											
Agree											
% Agree											

Interaction Skills Checklist

Parent: _____   Date ____ / ____ / ____   Time: ____

Child: _____   Observer: _____ (P R)

Setting/Activity: _____   Condition: Bl   Trtmt   Follow-up

\+ Completed correctly
– Completed incorrectly or not completed
N/A Not applicable

Parent Behaviors

Leveling	
Attending	
Appropriate touch	
Appropriate verbalizations	
Instructions	
Incidental teaching	

Child Behaviors

Appropriate verbalizations	
Affect	
Aggression	
Following instructions	

Example Activity Cards

During PCI training, parents are provided with a set of Activity Cards to keep. These 5" × 7" laminated cards show a picture of a parent and child engaging in the activity and have simple instructions. There is a set of approximately 12 activities for every age group. Each activity is age appropriate, and the instructions provide strategies for incorporating positive interactions between parents and children. Some activities are daily living activities, and others are activities that can take place at any time and do not require any supplies. Other activities require some planning and supplies.

Getting Dressed

- Try to help your child dress by him- or herself.
- Give your child a choice of clothing items ("Do you want the blue or the red shirt?")
- Ask your child where his or her body parts are before putting on clothing ("Show me your *arm*").
- Name pieces of clothing as you put them on.
- Talk about the color of the clothes.
- Talk about the right type of clothing for the weather. ("It's cold outside. We should wear sweaters.")
- Talk about the texture of the clothing (soft, rough, thick, thin).

Bath Time

- Have all of your supplies before you start (soap, shampoo, washcloth, towel, clothing, etc.).
- Talk about body parts.
- Sing bathtub songs ("Row, row, row your boat" or "Rubber Duckie").
- Smile and make eye contact with your child.
- Have bath toys available and talk about them as you bathe your child.

Finger Painting

Materials:

- Finger paints
- Paper
- Smock or clothing the child can get dirty

Suggestions:

- Set up the activity in a place where paint will not ruin anything, such as in the backyard or at the kitchen table with a plastic tablecloth on the table.
- Have your child feel the texture of the paint with his or her fingers.
- Talk about the colors.
- Mix paints together to make new colors (yellow and blue make green).
- Make handprints.
- Draw shapes or objects and guess what they are.

What Is On, Under, In, or Behind

- Ask questions about what items are inside another object, on top of another object, behind another object, and so forth.
- What is under the coffee table?

(continued)

- What is on top of the TV?
- Who is sitting in Mommy's chair?
- What is in the blue box?
- Take turns asking these questions of each other.

Storytelling

- Start a story with a few lines.
- Take turns adding one or two new lines to the story.
- Make up funny new characters.
- Tell stories that incorporate funny situations or things you have done with the child in the past.

Picture Album

This activity involves some preparation time, but older children can help.

- Cut out a variety of small pictures of interesting objects, people, and places from magazines.
- Glue the pictures to index cards or construction paper. You may also laminate them to make them last longer.
- When the cards are complete, talk about the pictures.
- Describe what you see in the pictures.(i.e., "I see kids playing"; "Here is a picture of a mother and her baby").
- Ask questions about the pictures (i.e., "Can you show me the horse?"; "How many ducks are there?"; "What is the woman doing?"; or "What color is the car?")
- Expand on what your child says (i.e., "That's right. That is a horse"; "There are three yellow ducks"; "She is mopping the floor"; "Yes, that is a blue car")
- Make up stories about the pictures.
- Sort the pictures according to categories (i.e., people, animals, food, etc.)

Dress Up

- Collect several different types of old clothing, such as shirts, hats, shoes, gloves, and so forth. (Check to be sure there is nothing in the pockets and that there are no loose buttons.)
- Play "dress up" and pretend to be different people.
- Talk about the different characters.
- Make up funny outfits and "model" these outfits for everyone.

Kitchen Play

This can be done during playtime and while parents are working in the kitchen, as long as the parent is closely supervising the child and there are safety latches on cupboards and drawers the child should not be in. Be sure that everything that the child can find is safe.

- Clean out a lower drawer or cupboard in the kitchen.
- Place a variety of plastic containers, lids, spoons, and lightweight pots or pans in this cupboard.
- Allow children to take these items out of this cupboard or drawer.
- Help your child stack containers, place lids on containers, or put containers inside larger containers.
- Use plastic spoons to pretend to mix food and cook.

(continued)

- Talk about the sizes of the containers and how some are heavy and some are light.
- Talk about the food you are pretending to cook.
- Allow the child to play with these items independently, but with your supervision, while you are cooking.

Play dough: Here is a recipe for play dough. This is an easy recipe to follow, and you can easily make this at home.

1 cup flour
½ cup salt
½ cup cooking oil
2 tablespoons of water
1 tablespoon of cream of tartar
You can add food coloring for color.
Mix everything together and you are ready.

- Talk about the feel of the play dough.
- Ask the child what he or she is building. If your child is young, do not ask the child to build a particular item, as this may be too difficult.
- Make shapes out of the play dough.
- Make similar shapes of different sizes and talk about the sizes of the shapes. Talk about the colors of the play dough, if you have used different colors of food coloring.

Planned Activities Training Checklist: Encouraging Independent Play When You Are Necessarily Busy

Parent: _____   Date ____ / ____ / ____ Time: ____

Child: _____   Observer: _____ (P R)

Setting/Activity: _____   Condition: Bl   Trtmt   Follow-up

+ Completed correctly
– Completed incorrectly or not completed
N/A Not applicable

Prepare in advance
      Get supplies ready in advance
      Have a plan for what you are going to do	

Enthusiastically help your child get started
      Select engaging and desired activities with your child
      Use incidental teaching	

Explain the rules for when you will be gone Simple, clear, and easy to follow	

Let the child know when you will return
      Anticipate interrupting your activity to check on your child
            periodically
      Select a short period of time so your child is sure to succeed	

Explain the rewards for following the rules Choice of activities, materials, where to play	
Set the timer Select a short period of time so your child is sure to succeed	

Interrupt your activity to praise your child
      In the beginning, check on your child often
      Be positive, and try to catch your child being good	

Ignore minor misbehavior
      Know what behaviors can be ignored and what need your
            attention	

Handle disruptions If possible, redirect your child to an activity and start again	

(continued)

When timer goes off, return to the child Be sure to follow up by returning when you said you would	
Explain to your child how he or she did	
Spend individual time with your child	
Percent correct:	

Parent–Child Interaction Training Consumer Satisfaction Questionnaire

Thank you for participating in the Parent–Child Interaction training offered by Project SafeCare. We would like to learn some of your thoughts and feelings about this program. Information we receive from parents like you will be used to improve the program and its effectiveness. Please read the following comments and circle the answer that best describes your feelings about each statement. Be as honest as possible, as your responses will not affect your interactions with Project SafeCare or other agencies. A space has been provided for you to add additional comments. Thank you for your time and cooperation.

1. The parent–child interactions program has improved my relationship with my child.

| Strongly agree | Agree | Neutral | Disagree | Strongly disagree |
| 1 | 2 | 3 | 4 | 5 |

2. I feel more patience toward my child.

| Strongly agree | Agree | Neutral | Disagree | Strongly disagree |
| 1 | 2 | 3 | 4 | 5 |

3. I enjoy the time I spend with my child more than before the training.

| Strongly agree | Agree | Neutral | Disagree | Strongly disagree |
| 1 | 2 | 3 | 4 | 5 |

4. My child's behavior has *not* improved since training in this component.

| Strongly agree | Agree | Neutral | Disagree | Strongly disagree |
| 1 | 2 | 3 | 4 | 5 |

5. I would recommend the Parent–Child Interaction program to other parents.

| Strongly agree | Agree | Neutral | Disagree | Strongly disagree |
| 1 | 2 | 3 | 4 | 5 |

6. The Parent–Child Interaction program has *not* changed the way I interact with my child(ren).

| Strongly agree | Agree | Neutral | Disagree | Strongly disagree |
| 1 | 2 | 3 | 4 | 5 |

Rate how useful each of these items was in helping you benefit from the services you received, if relevant.

	Useful	Somewhat useful	OK	Slightly useful	Useless
1. Counselor's explanations					
2. Counselor's demonstrations					
3. Practice during sessions					

(continued)

	Useful	Somewhat useful	OK	Slightly useful	Useless
4. Practice outside of sessions					
5. Counselor's feedback					
6. Written checklists					

Please rate the counselor who conducted the Parent–Child Interaction training program.

	Strongly agree	Agree	Neutral	Disagree	Strongly disagree
1. Was warm and friendly					
2. Was helpful					
3. Gave clear explanations					
4. Was knowledgeable					
5. Was negative or critical					
6. Treated me fairly					
7. Was willing to spend extra time when I needed it					
8. Kept our scheduled appointments					
9. Was on time to scheduled appointments					
10. Interacted well with my child					

Comments:

Recording Audiotapes for Use with Interval Recording Procedures

Materials: A blank audiotape of at least 20 minutes in length on one side, a tape recorder, and a stopwatch or clock with a second hand.

Script: Here is an example of what you will be recording:

> "This is a 10-second-observe, 5-second-record interval recording tape.
> Observe 1 . . . (wait 10 seconds) . . . Record 1 . . . (wait 5 seconds) . . .
> Observe 2 . . . (wait 10 seconds) . . . Record 2 . . . (wait 5 seconds) . . .
> Observe 3 . . . (wait 10 seconds) . . . Record 3 . . . (wait 5 seconds) . . . "

Instructions: To record a tape that can be used for a 10-minute observation, you will need to record prompts for 40 intervals (4 intervals per minute). Start by recording an introduction to the tape, so listeners are alerted to when the recording will begin.

When the second hand touches the "12," say "Observe 1." Wait for 10 seconds. When it touches the "2," say "Record 1." Wait for 5 seconds. When the second hand touches the "3," say "Observe 2." When it touches the 5, say "Record 2."

Continue recording 10-second-observe intervals and 5-second-record intervals while watching the second hand very closely. Be consistent when you begin saying each cue. For example, always begin saying either "observe" or "record" immediately as the second hand touches the appropriate point on the watch.

5

Planned Activities and Parent–Child Interaction Training

As described in Chapter 4, the rationale for Planned Activities Training (PAT) is that prevention is better than a cure. Parents are taught to promote appropriate and positive interactions with their children and to prevent challenging child behaviors. This component involves teaching parents to plan activities in advance, to prepare the child for these activities, and to engage the child in these activities. By doing so, parents can prevent challenging child behaviors, and the parent and child are able to enjoy increasingly positive interactions and activities.

The specific skills taught to parents in this component include acquiring basic parent–child interaction skills, preparing in advance, explaining rules and activities, selecting and engaging children in activities, using incidental teaching, and selecting and using reinforcers. Parent–Child Interaction training (PCI) and PAT are combined, and training can be adjusted so as to spend more time on the areas in which parents need more assistance. For example, if parents' interaction skills (quality of verbalizations, touch, instructions, etc.) are acceptable but their use of strategies for preventing challenging behavior are in need of improvement, more time should be spent conducting PAT, which addresses this need.

Depending on the level of instruction the parent may require before observing and practicing the skills, and if there are many other children present, it may be helpful for a second counselor to take other children (i.e., those children who will not participate in the training session) to another room or at least to occupy them in an activity nearby.

GENERAL SESSION FORMAT FOR PARENT TRAINING PROTOCOL

Each training session, which lasts 1½ to 2 hours (five sessions), incorporates the following general elements: instructions with rationale, modeling, practice, and feedback. A general outline for each training session is provided later, but the following steps are those that should be followed during each training session when teaching or practicing a specific behavior or skill. (Table 5.1 provides an overview of the general training protocol for each session; Table 5.2 provides a concise overview of each parent training session.)

I. Explain target behaviors.
   A. Identify the behaviors to be trained in the session.
   B. Describe each behavior (see assessment protocol for operational definitions and examples).
   C. Provide a rationale for each behavior.
   D. Describe examples or applications of behavior.
   E. Ask for and answer parent's questions.
   F. Encourage and praise parent's suggestions and ideas.
II. Model each behavior
   A. Demonstrate the target behavior in normal setting or situation.
   B. *Keep demonstration simple*.
   C. Ask parent to observe and identify each behavior.
III. Parent practice
   A. Ask parent to practice each behavior.
   B. Check off steps of PAT demonstrated correctly using the PAT checklist (and a checklist of interaction skills, if this is being used).
   C. Take notes regarding specific skills that are performed well and skills that are in need of more practice.
IV. Feedback
   A. Use the PAT checklist, interaction skills checklist (if applicable), and notes to provide descriptive feedback.
   B. Feedback should always be delivered in a positive and descriptive manner. Even when parents have not demonstrated any of the steps correctly, praise any aspect of the interaction that approximated the desired performance. *For example, praise the parent's tone of voice, the choice of activity in which they engaged their child, or their making eye contact with the child.*

TABLE 5.1. General Session Format for Planned Activities and Parent–Child Interaction Training

1. Explain desired target behavior.
2. Describe and model each behavior.
3. Ask parent to practice behavior; observe with checklist.
4. Give parent positive feedback for correct behaviors; describe and model behaviors needing more practice.
5. Ask parent to practice behaviors; observe with checklist.
6. Review parent performance and set goals/homework for coming week.
7. Review and end the session.

TABLE 5.2. Planned Activities and Parent–Child Interactions Training Sessions

Session 1

I. Establish an agenda.
II. Conduct assessment observation of parent and child interaction in a play situation or other problematic situation.
III. Review progress.
IV. Identify problem settings.
V. Provide rationale for PAT.
VI. Describe, model, and give feedback on parent–child interaction skills.
VII. Provide a set of activity cards to parents.
VIII. Describe how to prepare in advance by organizing and managing time more effectively.
IX. Describe how to explain the activity, the rules, and the consequences regarding desired and undesired behavior in a relaxed and noncoercive manner.
X. Explain how to provide engaging and stimulating activities for children in specific home and community settings.
XI. Describe how to encourage and extend children's engagement in activities by use of incidental teaching.
XII. Discuss how to select and apply practical procedures for motivating children's behavior in different settings (using good interaction skills).
XIII. Discuss providing rewards and practical consequences.
XIV. Demonstrate giving children feedback following the activity.
XV. Summary

Session 2

I. Establish an agenda.
II. Conduct observation of parent and child activity, providing positive feedback on correct skills use, modeling if necessary, and suggesting additional practice for incorrectly demonstrated skills.
III. Review progress since previous session.
IV. Model PAT checklists in a home setting.
V. Model checklist for community setting.
VI. Establish goals.
VII. Summary

Session 3

I. Establish an agenda.
II. Conduct observation of parent and child activity, providing positive feedback on correct skills use, modeling if necessary, and suggesting additional practice for incorrectly demonstrated skills.
III. Review progress since previous session.
IV. Model PAT checklists in a home setting.
V. Model checklist for community setting.
VI. Establish goals.
VII. Summary

Session 4

I. Establish an agenda.
II. Conduct observation of parent and child activity, providing positive feedback on correct skills use, modeling if necessary, and suggesting additional practice for incorrectly demonstrated skills.
III. Practice encouraging independent play when parents are busy.
IV. Establish goals.
V. Summary

(continued)

TABLE 5.2. *(continued)*

Session 5

   I. Establish an agenda.

  II. Conduct observation of parent and child activity, providing positive feedback on correct skills use, modeling if necessary, and suggesting additional practice for incorrectly demonstrated skills.

 III. Practice encouraging independent play when parents are busy.

 IV. Independent future problem solving.

  V. Summary

     C. Provide feedback in the following manner:

       1. Provide overall, evaluative statement (positive emphasis).

       2. Provide two to three examples of behaviors parent performed well. *Note:* Even if parent did not perform target behaviors well, first provide feedback on any aspect of the interaction that *was* performed well.

       3. Describe behaviors that parent should focus on when practicing. Maintain positive emphasis. Point out one to two skills the parent should practice. Review the behaviors to be practiced.

  V. Additional practice

     A. Ask parent to demonstrate at least two more times any steps not practiced correctly. You might also ask parent to practice doing it a little differently each time, introducing natural variations into the interaction.

     B. Prompt parent to continue to practice target behaviors.

     C. Observe performance and make note of the steps or behaviors demonstrated correctly.

     D. Give feedback on practice attempt (as described in section IV).

 VI. Review performance.

     A. After practice trials, identify behaviors parent should continue to practice before next session.

     B. Leave a prompt with the parent, such as a PAT checklist or clearly written notes.

     C. Agree on the number of activities the parent and child are to engage in before the next session. The counselor should suggest a reasonable number of activities per day and should remind the parent that he or she can practice in any situation that occurs throughout the week.

     D. Give clear description of assignment. For example, "In the following week, I would like you to practice PAT during bath time with your child. Next time I visit, we will practice these again so you can show me how well you are doing."

     E. Leave with the parent a data sheet to record activities and the activity cards.

VII. Review the session.

     A. Review the behaviors targeted in the session.

     B. Review the parent's performance during the practice trials.

     C. Include behaviors performed well and those that the parent should continue to practice.

     D. Review the "homework assignment" for the next session.

    E. Use additional teaching strategies as necessary.
       1. Ask parent to give feedback about counselor's performance of target behaviors, using the PAT checklists.
       2. Ask parent to observe a secondary counselor perform target behaviors.
       3. If two parents are participating in training *and* marital or partner conflict is not an issue, have them give feedback to each other.
       4. Interact with child, and have parent prompt counselor to perform target behaviors as appropriate.
    Note: Be sure to record the teaching strategies used on the data sheet and in the case notes.

TRAINING SITUATIONS

In Project SafeCare, training was always conducted during standard situations common to most parent–child interactions. Generally, training took place during playtime and during two daily living activities, such as mealtime, bath time, dressing, and bedtime. When working with individual families, training can be conducted in any situation that poses difficulties for the family.

In order to assess generalization, which is the transfer of skills learned in one situation to a new, untrained situation, observations may be conducted in situations in which training has not been provided. For example, if training is provided during playtime, grocery shopping, and bath time, the counselor might ask the parents to demonstrate their use of PAT during mealtime in order to assess the generalization of PAT to this novel situation.

MASTERY CRITERION

Although the training procedures are described in five discrete sessions, training should be tailored to the parent's performance. Mastery criterion for PAT is 100% of the steps demonstrated correctly. That is, when the parent has demonstrated 100% of the steps of a specific activity checklist correctly, then they have mastered PAT in that activity. If the 100% criterion is not met during the initial session in which an activity is introduced, practice during subsequent training sessions should continue until the parent meets this criterion. This may involve revising the procedures slightly to allow time for additional practice, while providing training in a variety of situations.

TRAINING PROCEDURES

Session 1

    I. Establish an agenda.
      A. Greet the parent and take care of any other business. Explain what will occur during this session.

B. Explain that, first you will help the family determine which situations are trouble-some. Then you will observe the parent and child interacting during an activity. Next you will explain PAT, demonstrate PAT with the child, and ask the parent to practice PAT in the same situation in which you demonstrated it. Following prac-tice, you will give feedback and help the parent master each of the following steps of PAT: preparing in advance, explaining the activity, explaining the rules, explain-ing the consequences, giving choices, talking about what they are doing, using good interaction skills, ignoring minor misbehavior, giving feedback, and providing re-wards or consequences. *Note*: Depending on the skill level of the parent, determine whether it will be more beneficial for the parent to observe and practice each skill one at a time or whether the parent will be able to observe an entire interaction and then practice all of the steps at one time in an interaction. Then structure each training session appropriately. This involves determining how many skills the coun-selor demonstrates at one time and how many steps the parent is asked to practice.

C. Throughout training, which takes place in approximately five sessions, there will be opportunities to modify the PAT steps as needed. *Note*: In Project SafeCare, train-ing generally took place during a few standard situations, such as playtime, meal-time, bath time, dressing, and bedtime (see Appendices 4.3–4.7 in Chapter 4). Training in PAT can be conducted in any situation that the family finds problem-atic. Additional PAT checklists may be obtained from the authors.

II. Conduct assessment observation of parent and child interaction in a play situation or other problematic situation.

A. Initial modeling and practice takes place during a play situation that is easily set up during the session. For example, the counselor might bring a game or puzzle with him or her to use during modeling and practice, or the parent might suggest an ap-propriate play activity that the child enjoys.

III. Review progress.

A. Changes may have occurred during the assessment process. Invite parents to com-ment on how they view progress. Prompt parents to identify any positive or nega-tive changes in their child's behavior. If there are decreases or increases in chal-lenging behavior, ask about changes in routine that may have prompted these changes.

IV. Identify problem settings.

A. Invite parents to identify settings in which they are experiencing problems or have them fill out a Daily Activities Checklist. Present a brief summary of PAT, interac-tion skill data, and anecdotal information gathered from assessment observations to the parents and decide on situations in which training should be conducted. First describe the many positive aspects that were observed in the interaction. For exam-ple, you might say,

> "I really liked the way you talked about and named body parts while you were dressing Jack. I also liked the way you were positive and provided praise for his cooperation during bath time."

Then describe the areas in which the parent can improve his or her interactions. For example, you might say,

> "Next time, you might try explaining to Sarah where you will be going and what the rules are before you go out to do errands. She will have a better understanding of what to expect and what is expected of her, as well as what the rewards will be for following the rules."

Generally, training should be conducted in at least three situations. In Project SafeCare, training was conducted primarily in home situations, but PAT can be conducted in any home or community settings. By conducting training in more than one situation and by including situations that are diverse, the likelihood increases that parents' skills will generalize to novel situations in which training was not conducted.

    B. Decide on the setting in which training will first be conducted. Generally, the activity in which there is a need for change and in which the parents can achieve success is the best activity in which to begin training. Then, as parents meet the mastery criterion for these situations, more challenging situations may be introduced.

  V. Provide rationale for PAT.

    A. Mention that you will now begin to discuss ways of dealing with the child's behavior in the settings mentioned.

    B. Outline the basic ideas underlying PAT.

      1. The primary objective of PAT is prevention of challenging behavior. If situations can be arranged so that misbehavior does not occur, then parents do not need to worry about dealing with challenging behavior.

      2. Encouraging children to be involved in activities reduces the opportunity for misbehavior. When children are engaged in activities, they are less likely to misbehave.

 VI. Describe, model, and give feedback on parent–child interaction skills.

    A. Describe each parent interaction skill and give examples of its use. Parent behaviors include leveling, attending, touch, verbalizations, instructions, and incidental teaching (see Chapter 4 for definitions).

    B. Model skills for parent as necessary. Ask parent to practice those skills that were not demonstrated during assessment observations.

    C. Provide positive and corrective feedback and then ask parent to continue to practice until the skill is demonstrated correctly. If additional practice is needed, explain that there will be several opportunities to practice throughout the training sessions.

VII. Provide a set of activity cards to parents (see Appendix 4.10 in Chapter 4 for sample cards).

    A. Describe the rationale for activity cards. They provide suggestions for simple, age-appropriate activities in which the parent and child can interact. By interacting in enriching and stimulating activities with their children, they are teaching valuable skills.

       B. *Parents may keep these activity cards to prompt them to engage in activities with their children after training is complete.*

       C. Explain that you will model interacting with the child in some of these activities later in training.

  VIII. Describe how to prepare in advance by organizing and managing time more effectively.

       A. Discuss issues related to organizing time to avoid last-minute rushing and panic situations. Invite parents to make changes in their schedules to provide time to hold a discussion with the child before the PAT situation.

       B. Parents are reinforced naturally for planning to avoid problems. Having the right supplies at hand, having a simple schedule for the day, and being prepared for surprises can help prevent problems.

       C. Discuss strategies for being prepared that are specific to situations the parent faces on a regular basis.

    IX. Describe how to explain the activity, the rules, and the consequences regarding desired and undesired behavior in a relaxed and noncoercive manner.

       A. After gaining the child's attention, the parent should explain the activity and why that activity is taking place. For example, "We are going to the grocery store because we need milk for your cereal."

       B. As counselor, you should model appropriate discussion skills that involve the child in the establishment of a rule. Explain that parent should:

          1. Always explain to children what will be happening next and what the rules are for the activity.

          2. Use positive interaction skills while explaining rules.

          3. Keep rules clear, simple, reasonable, and enforceable.
            Examples:

- "Keep your hands to yourself."
- "Use an 'inside' voice."
- "Keep the play dough on the table."
- "Wash your hands after going to the bathroom."
- "Keep your food on your plate."
- "Wipe your mouth with a napkin."
- "Touch your baby sister softly."
- "Stay with Mom while you are in the store."
- "Hold Dad's hand while we cross the street."
- "Put your toys on the shelf when you are done playing."

          4. Tell the child the rules and explain the reasons for them. Try to frame the rules in the positive rather than the negative. For example, "Don't touch" should be stated as "Keep your hands to yourself." "Don't yell" becomes "use an 'indoor' voice."

          5. Tell the child the consequence for breaking the rules. "If you cannot keep your bottom on the chair, then you will have to get down from the table," or "If you

don't keep the game pieces on the table, then we will have to put the game away."

6. Tell the child the consequences for following the rules. For example, "If you go to bed on time, then we will read a story together," or "If you keep your hands to yourself in the grocery store, you can pick out a cereal."

7. Be willing and able to carry out the consequences he or she describes to the child. Further, consequences should be delivered as soon after the appropriate behavior as possible.

8. Check to be sure that the child heard and understood the rules by asking what the rules are and having the child repeat the rules.

C. Have the parent identify what he or she noticed about the interaction and identify its impact on the child.

D. Ask the parent to model the discussion.

E. Provide feedback. Ask parent to practice again any steps not demonstrated correctly.

X. Explain how to provide engaging and stimulating activities for children in specific home and community settings.

A. Introduce concept of engagement. When children are busy, they are less disruptive.

B. Provide examples of activities that can be used when in the car, shopping, or visiting. Some of these examples may be depicted on Activity Cards.

C. Have parent add additional activities to the list. Keep in mind specific activities that are preferred by the child and also activities that would be appropriate in a variety of settings, such as the doctor's office, in the car, or while the parent is preparing a meal.

XI. Describe how to encourage and extend children's engagement in activities by use of incidental teaching.

A. Having activities available is no guarantee children will play with them. The goal here is to make interactions with toys and tasks more reinforcing and rewarding for the child.

B. Introduce incidental teaching as a way of increasing child's interest in an activity.

1. Incidental teaching is a simple way of engaging children in activities, teaching simple skills, and encouraging language development.

2. Throughout the day, there are numerous opportunities for engaging in incidental teaching in naturally occurring situations.

3. The basic principle is to observe and talk with children about the activities in which they are demonstrating interest. This can be done in a number of ways, such as describing what the child is doing, elaborating on the child's activities, providing suggestions for ways of expanding on the activity, or asking questions about the activity.

4. If the parent is not sure what the child is interested in, he or she should ask questions, such as "What are you doing?"

5. If the child does not become engaged in the conversation, parents can gently prompt the child to answer questions or talk about the activity. For example, if

the child does not answer the question "What color is that?" the parent can simply say, "That's blue." It is important that these interactions are fun and positive.

6. One rule is to always follow the child's lead. The parent should not try to direct the activity or insist that the child "learn something" from the activity. Interactions should always be positive, fun, and enriching.

7. If the parent becomes agitated or angry or the child loses interest, the interaction should be terminated, or they should be redirected to another activity.

C. Demonstrate incidental teaching during an activity in which the child is engaged.

D. Prompt parents to comment on what they noticed.

E. Have the parent role play using incidental teaching, and provide feedback.

F. Discuss novelty. Encourage parents to introduce a new activity before the child becomes bored with the old one and to reinforce the child's engagement in activity with attention.

XII. Discuss how to select and apply practical procedures for motivating children's behavior in different settings (using good interaction skills).

A. Prompt parents to identify possible natural and tangible rewards.

B. Brainstorm with the parent about activities, toys, items, places, foods, and people that the child prefers. These may be activities that the child currently engages in or asks for or novel activities. Make a list of all the ideas for rewards. Provide these things for children during activities as a way of engaging children and rewards for desired behavior.

C. Remind the parent that rewards do not always need to be food items or things that they must buy for their child. Often, attention and fun activities are the best rewards.

D. Rewards should be delivered as quickly as possible.

E. When rewards cannot be delivered immediately, remind parents to offer praise and tell the child what he or she has earned and will get later. For example, after the child has shown good behavior while doing errands, the parent might tell the child, "You did a great job following the rules. When we get home, we'll have time to walk to the park before dinner."

XIII. Discuss providing rewards and practical consequences.

A. Explain to parent that consequences are not a primary focus of PAT. The primary objective is arranging the child's environment so that he or she is engaged and building new skills. Thus artificial consequences are less relevant. Sometimes, however, regardless of our efforts to prevent challenging behavior, it still occurs.

B. Discuss ignoring minor misbehavior and using terminating instructions. Parents feel more confident if they know how to handle challenging behavior.

1. Discuss giving instructions to "stop" or "listen" or to attend to some other event. For example, if the child is about to run while crossing the street, the parent might say, "Stop running, come here and hold my hand."

2. Explain that instructions should be given in a similar manner to which rules are given. They should be simple, clear, stated positively, and easy to follow.

3. Tell parent that minor misbehavior can be ignored in many cases. Parents should decide which behaviors are minor and can be ignored.

    4. Explain how to redirect the child into an activity using incidental teaching.

  C. Prompt parents to use these strategies and to stick with their current method of dealing with problems.

XIV. Demonstrate giving children feedback following the activity.

  A. Model how to hold a discussion with the child following an activity and to provide constructive feedback on desirable and less desirable behavior.

    1. Tell the child what he or she did well, such as, "You did a wonderful job staying with me at the grocery store. Thank you so much."

    2. Tell the child what he or she needs to improve next time. For example, "Next time, remember to use a quiet voice while we are in the library."

    3. Check that children remember by asking what they did well and what they need to improve.

    4. Follow through with rewards for following the rules and consequences for breaking the rules. For example, "You cannot go to the park because you did not keep your hands to yourself at the store. If you help me clean up your toys when we get home, then you can watch your favorite video."

  B. Have parent comment on what he or she observed.

  C. Have parent practice, and give feedback.

XV. Summary

  A. Summarize the content of the session and answer any of the parent's questions.

  B. Provides parents with written summary to read before the next session. This might include handwritten notes specific to the family or general PAT checklists.

  C. Decide with the parent on activities in which parent will begin to practice PAT. Ask the parent to practice using PAT during these activities.

  D. Decide with the parent which activity cards the parent and child will use during the following week.

  E. Explain that, during the next session, you will ask the parent and child to engage in an activity in order to observe the parent's use of PAT and that they will continue to practice using PAT in a variety of situations.

Session 2

  I. Establish an agenda.

  A. Outline what will be covered in the session.

    1. First, you will observe the parent and child engaging in an activity in order to find out how PAT is working for them at this point. Then, you and the parent will review the skills discussed at the previous session.

    2. Explain that during this session there will be opportunities for additional practice using PAT in different activities.

  II. Conduct an observation of parent–child interactions in order to assess parent's use of PAT and the parent's and the child's interaction skills. Refer to the section on Conducting Observations (see Chapter 4 for instruction). Provide feedback on skills demonstrated correctly, and ask parents to practice again the skills demonstrated incorrectly. Provide additional instructions and modeling as necessary.

III. Review progress since previous session
   A. Discuss parent's practice during the previous week and the results. Ask parent to describe the situations in which PAT was practiced and the effects on parent–child interactions and child behavior.
   B. Answer parent's questions.
IV. Model PAT checklists in a home setting
   A. Select one home setting or situation that has been problematic for the family.
   B. Give the parent the PAT checklist for that setting (either a preprinted one or one written specifically for that family) and discuss each step. Be sure to write down and discuss information specific to the family, including specific rules, activities, and reinforcers.
   C. Answer parent's questions.
   D. Model PAT in that activity for the parent. Involve the child in the activity, using all steps described on the PAT checklist. Ask the parent to follow along while looking at her or his copy of the checklist. Tell her or him to check each step off as you demonstrate it.
   E. Ask the parent to practice engaging the child in that same activity, following the steps listed on the checklist. If the activity is one that can easily be repeated, the parent should engage in the series of steps in that activity after you finish demonstrating them. If the step is not easily repeated, such as a meal or bath, ask the parent to practice each step following you at appropriate times throughout the activity. For example, during mealtime, you should model explaining the rules and consequences before the meal, and the parent should practice those steps at that time, rather than when mealtime is complete.
   F. Provide feedback to parent either during the activity or at the end, whichever is appropriate. Provide positive feedback on the skills the parent demonstrated well and then offer corrective feedback on the skills that can be improved. Provide additional instruction and modeling as needed. Ask parents to practice again the steps that were not completed correctly.
V. Model checklist for community setting
   A. Select a community setting that has been problematic for the family. *Note*: In Project SafeCare, training primarily took place in the home and not in community settings. In order to promote maintenance and generalization, it is best to provide training in the settings in which problems are most likely to occur. In some cases, it will be important to go out to community settings with the family in order to teach PAT. For example, rather than meeting at the family's home, you might go with the family to the grocery store and model and practice PAT during a shopping trip. In this situation, counselor modeling and parent practice would take place in the same fashion as during home visits.
   B. Give the parent the PAT checklist (or construct one together with the parent) for that setting and discuss each step as it would be carried out in the community. If you are conducting the session in the community, model each step of the checklist.
   C. Ask the parent to practice, and then provide feedback on parent performance. When appropriate in a community setting, ask the parent to practice again any steps not completed correctly.

       D. Answer the parent's questions.

       E. Explain that similar checklists are available for other home and community settings.

  VI. Establish goals

       A. Ask the parent to implement PAT in the home setting in which practice took place and in the community setting that was discussed or visited.

       B. With the parent, determine activities during which PAT practice will take place during the upcoming week.

       C. You and the parent should also decide which activity cards the parent and child will use during the following week.

       4. Tell the parent that you will review these practice sessions at your next meeting.

 VII. Summary

       A. Review main points discussed during this session.

       B. Answer any questions.

Session 3

   I. Establish an agenda

       A. Outline what will be covered in the session.

          1. First, you will observe the parent and child engaging in an activity in order to find out how PAT is working for them at this point. Then you and the parent will review the skills discussed at the previous session.

          2. Explain that during this session there will be opportunities for additional practice using PAT in different activities.

  II. Conduct an observation of the parent and child engaging in an activity in order to observe parent's use of PAT and the parent's and the child's interaction skills. Refer to the section on Conducting Observations (see Chapter 4 for instructions). Provide feedback on skills demonstrated correctly, and ask parents to practice again the skills demonstrated incorrectly. Provide additional instructions and modeling as necessary.

 III. Review progress since previous session

       A. Discuss parent's practice during the previous week and the results. Ask parent to describe the situations in which PAT was practiced and the effects on parent–child interactions and child behavior.

       B. Answer parent's questions.

 IV. Model PAT Checklists in a home setting

       A. Select one novel home setting or situation that has been problematic for the family, or continue practicing a situation that is still problematic for the family.

       B. Give the parent the PAT checklist for that setting (either a preprinted one or one written specifically for that family) and discuss each step. Be sure to write down and discuss information specific to the family, including specific rules, activities, and reinforcers.

       C. Answer parent's questions.

       D. Model PAT in that activity for the parent. Involve the child in the activity, using all steps described on the PAT checklist. Ask the parent to follow along while looking at her or his copy of the checklist. Tell her or him to check each step off as you demonstrate it.

E. Ask the parent to practice engaging the child in that same activity, following the steps listed on the checklist. If the activity is one that can easily be repeated, the parent should engage in the series of steps in that activity after you finish demonstrating them. If the step is not easily repeated, such as a meal or bath, ask the parent to practice each step following you at appropriate times throughout the activity. For example, during mealtime, you should model explaining the rules and consequences before the meal, and the parent should practice those steps at that time, rather than when mealtime is complete.

F. As training progresses and parents demonstrate skills at criterion level, which is 100% of the appropriate PAT steps on a checklist, the level of prompting and modeling you need to do should decrease. You should discriminate the steps that parents demonstrate at criterion level from the steps that the parent still needs to practice and provide modeling and prompting only for those skills that the parent has not yet mastered. Special attention should be paid to those skills that engage the child in activities, thus preventing challenging behavior. For example, during all activities, parents should be encouraged to use incidental teaching as a strategy for teaching skills, encouraging language use and development, and engaging the child in the current activity.

G. Provide feedback to parent either during the activity or at the end, whichever is appropriate. Again, the feedback should include positive comments for skills demonstrated correctly and corrective comments for those steps that are not yet demonstrated at criterion level.

V. Model checklist for community setting

A. Select a community setting that has been problematic for the family.

B. Give the parent the PAT checklist (or construct one together with the parent) for that setting and discuss each step as it would be carried out in the community. If you are conducting the session in the community, model each step of the checklist.

C. Ask the parent to practice, and then provide feedback on parent performance. When appropriate in a community setting, ask the parent to practice again any steps not completed correctly.

D. Answer the parent's questions.

E. Explain that similar checklists are available for other home and community settings.

VI. Establish goals

A. Ask the parent to implement PAT in the settings in which practice took place.

B. With the parent, determine activities during which PAT practice will take place during the upcoming week.

C. You and the parent should also decide which activity cards the parent and child will use during the following week.

D. Tell the parent that you will review these practice sessions at your next meeting.

VII. Summary

A. Review main points discussed during this session.

B. Answer any questions.

Session 4

I. Establish an agenda
   A. Outline what will be covered in the session
      1. First, you will observe the parent and child engaging in an activity in order to find out how PAT is working for them at this point. Then you and the parent will review the skills discussed at the previous session.
      2. Explain that during this session there will be opportunities for additional practice using PAT in different activities. Specifically, you will review the activities in which PAT was used during the previous week, including any new activities to which the parent has applied her or his new skills. You will also practice encouraging children to play independently while the parent is busy.
II. Conduct an observation of the parent and child engaging in an activity in order to observe parent's use of PAT and the parent's and the child's interaction skills. Refer to the section on Conducting Observations (see Chapter 4 for instructions). Provide feedback on skills demonstrated correctly, and ask parents to practice again the skills demonstrated incorrectly. Provide additional instructions and modeling as necessary.
III. Practice encouraging independent play when parents are busy
   A. Ask the parent to engage the child in an activity while the two of you talk. Provide the checklist titled "Encouraging Independent Play When You Are Necessarily Busy" (Appendix 4.11, Chapter 4).
   B. Prompt the parent to explain the rules to the child and to occasionally interrupt their conversation with you to praise the child.
   C. During this conversation, review the progress since the previous session. Assist parent in identifying solutions for problems the parent experienced.
IV. Establish goals
   A. Ask the parent to implement PAT in the settings in which practice took place.
   B. With the parent, determine activities during which PAT practice will take place during the upcoming week.
   C. You and the parent should also decide which activity cards the parent and child will use during the following week.
   D. Tell the parent that you will review these practice sessions at your next meeting.
V. Summary
   A. Review main points discussed during this session.
   B. Answer any questions.

Session 5

I. Establish an agenda
   A. Review progress.
   B. Practice encouraging independent play.
   C. Discuss problem-solving strategies to handle future problems.
II. Conduct an observation of the parent and child engaging in an activity in order to observe parent's use of PAT and the parent's and the child's interaction skills. Refer to the

section on Conducting Observations (see Chapter 4 for instructions). Provide feedback on skills demonstrated correctly, and ask parents to practice again the skills demonstrated incorrectly. Provide additional instructions and modeling as necessary.

III. Practice encouraging independent play when parents are busy
   A. Ask the parent to engage the child in an activity while the two of you talk. Provide the checklist titled "Encouraging Independent Play When You Are Necessarily Busy" (Appendix 4.11).
   B. Prompt the parent to explain the rules to the child and to occasionally interrupt their conversation with you to praise the child.
   C. During this conversation, review the progress since the previous session. Assist parent in identifying solutions for problems the parent experienced.

IV. Independent future problem solving
   A. Review basic steps for designing a PAT intervention.
   B. Prompt the parent to identify one remaining problem and one possible future problem.
   C. Give the parent a blank behavior checklist and ask her or him to design an intervention for these areas. Provide assistance only as needed.
   D. Ask parent to implement the program for the checklists she or he has developed, and remind the parent that she or he can now develop a plan to handle the situations that present themselves in the future.

V. Summary
   A. Ask parents to continue to review and practice PAT checklists.
   B. Summarize the key PAT steps and the progress the parent has made in implementing the steps.
   C. Remind the parent that using PAT will help engage children in activities, teach important skills, and decrease children's problem behavior.

CONSUMER SATISFACTION SURVEY

In order to assess parents' satisfaction with the training procedures and the results, you may ask parents to complete the Consumer Satisfaction Questionnaire (Appendix 4.12, Chapter 4). Inform parents that their feedback is highly valued and helps improve services provided to other parents.

COMMON PROBLEMS AND SOLUTIONS

PAT places a greater emphasis on positive interactions between parents and children and does not stress the use of consequences. Many parents value this aspect of PAT and indicate that using PAT seems very natural and comfortable. There are, however, some common problems that arise in teaching PAT. Frequently, parents may disagree over the use of rewards or reinforcers. Sometimes this may be due to the misperception that rewards must cost a great deal of money or that parents must offer sweets or snacks to children as rewards. Although in some cases, edible rewards or items costing some amount of money may be used as rewards, it is often the case that the most effective rewards may be a parent's attention or a special activity or privilege. For example, sitting down and having playtime with a favorite toy or game, reading a special book, watching a favorite video, or going for a walk can all be highly effective rewards. Outings to the park, visiting a friend or relative, helping Mom prepare lunch, or helping Dad rake leaves are all activities that can act as rewards. Some parents keep a few favorite toys packed away so that they can bring out this favorite item when a special reward is needed. If a child has not played with it for a couple of weeks, it becomes a highly desired item. For older children, art projects using items such as safety scissors, glue, glitter, and scraps of paper or pictures cut from magazines may be especially rewarding. In some cases, if it is not too cost prohibitive, parents may choose to purchase a special item for their child as a reward for good behavior. While grocery shopping, parents may allow the child to pick out a special cereal or snack or a small toy when they have followed the rules while shopping. Novelty is an important factor in selecting reinforcers. By varying the types of reinforcers provided to children, parents will optimize their effectiveness.

Another common problem that has been encountered in PAT is that parents may be uncomfortable role playing. It is important first to explain this aspect of the training protocol before actually doing any role playing, so that parents are aware of this expectation. Explaining that role playing is a key step in learning these new skills may help parents understand its importance. Acknowledge that it can seem very different and uncomfortable practicing new skills, especially in front of other people. Explain that we all experience this discomfort and that this feeling usually goes away as we become more familiar with and are better at using these new skills. You may also offer to play the role of the parent in some situations. Humor can also go a long way in reducing any fear about role playing.

Finally, cultural and language differences, as well as reading abilities, may make the implementation of PAT difficult. Whenever possible, it is important to try to match ethnicity and language between counselors and families. In some cases, cultural differences may lead to disagreement over particular aspects of PAT. For instance, as describe in the following case example, one family did not believe that children should talk much at the dinner table. Although the counselor explained that engaging in conversation during mealtime may make this time of day more rewarding for children, she ultimately left this choice to the parents, once she observed that the parents were engaging in very positive interactions at other times of the day with their child. Parents who have reading deficits may not be able to use the written materials, such as activity cards and PAT checklists, to a great extent, but this does not preclude the counselor from teaching these skills or using pictures to convey the message of some of these materials.

CASE EXAMPLE

The Lopez family was reported for child abuse. Mr. Lopez had been physically abusive to his 5-year-old son, Paul. Several observations were made of parent–child interactions during playtime, mealtime, and while the child was getting dressed. Mr. and Mrs. Lopez did not engage Paul in activities, so he was often indulging in undesirable behavior, such as not following instructions, not eating his food, being distracted by other activities, or dawdling while getting dressed. When his parents told him to eat his food or get dressed, Paul became resistant and had tantrums. These are the problems that appeared to prompt Mr. Lopez to use excessive physical punishment with his son. For these reasons, it was determined that PAT would be the appropriate form of training.

During the first training session, the counselor and the parents discussed the problems they experienced with Paul. The parents felt that Paul should be able to bathe and dress himself alone and to eat his meal quietly. The counselor discussed which responsibilities were reasonable to expect of a 5-year-old child and which were not. Then she described the steps of PAT. She also modeled each of these steps during a play activity. The parents checked off each step as they observed it during this activity.

The counselor then asked each of them to engage in a play activity with Paul using PAT, good interaction skills, and incidental teaching. In general, the parents used many of the steps of PAT, and the mother used good interaction skills. Specific instances of good uses of PAT and interaction skills were pointed out. The father did not talk to Paul or use incidental teaching, and thus the counselor gently provided corrective feedback on his verbal interaction skills and use of incidental teaching. It would have been inappropriate to provide more negative than positive feedback, so the counselor focused on helping Mr. Lopez increase the talk he directed toward his son. This, too, was accomplished through role playing and feedback. Additional feedback aimed at increasing the quality of those verbalizations and at refining their use of PAT and incidental teaching would take place during subsequent sessions. Additional modeling was provided in a variety of play activities. Although the parents were skeptical and felt as if Paul should "be good" without their extra effort, they agreed to try using PAT in the coming weeks. Several copies of the appropriate PAT checklists were left for the parents to refer to throughout the week. They were asked to check off each step they used during specific interactions so that they could discuss at the next meeting how these new strategies worked for them. They were also asked to make note of Paul's behavior in each of the interactions so that they could see how their new way of interacting with their son was affecting his behavior. The counselor reminded the parents that change might take place slowly and that it might be difficult or unnatural at first to use such different skills, but she reassured them that over time, things would get easier and Paul's behavior would improve if they consistently practiced.

Throughout the next four sessions, the parents and the counselor continued to discuss PAT, interaction skills, and incidental teaching, and, more important, the counselor provided a great deal of modeling, followed by parent practice and feedback. The parents practiced engaging Paul in play activities, as well as during mealtime, while he was getting ready for school in the morning, and during other various activities. They also practiced PAT while at the grocery store. The counselor continued to observe Mr. and Mrs. Lopez at each session, collecting data on their use of PAT, on their interaction skills, and on Paul's behavior. Feedback was always specific so that they could continue to practice those steps that had posed the greatest difficulty to them. When Mr. and Mrs. Lopez reached the 100% mastery criterion in a given activity, the counselor enthusiastically praised their efforts and then helped them select additional activities to which PAT could be applied. By the fifth session, Mrs. Lopez had reached the 100% mastery criterion for three different activities; Mr. Lopez had mastered two but had completed only 90% of the steps correctly for mealtime. The counselor explained that training would be complete when he had scored 100% on the mealtime PAT checklist. With this comment, however, Mr. Lopez explained that he did not feel that children should spend much time talking at the dinner table. He understood the importance of talking to his son during other activities but did not feel that there should be excessive talking during mealtime. This was understood to be a difference of opinion possibly due to differing expectations among diverse cultures. Because Mr. Lopez had already met the 100% mastery criterion in all of the other activities, the counselor thanked Mr. Lopez for his honesty, and training was concluded with a summary of the main components of PAT, interaction skills, and incidental teaching.

Then they discussed how what they had learned could be applied to problems they might encounter in the future as their son continues to grow and develop. Over the next few months, while other training components were completed, Mr. and Mrs. Lopez reported that they continued to notice improvements in Paul's behavior. In addition, they reported that they now enjoyed playing with Paul, and they felt that he was enjoying their interactions also.

Thus PAT is an extremely useful parent-training tool. Its focus is on *preventing* challenging behavior and on improving the parent–child bond.

ON DATA COLLECTION

The rigorous direct observation suggested here might seem cumbersome to those not familiar with doing it. In many cases, it also may not be possible. In defense of this approach, we argue that collecting systematic data based on direct observation and careful operational definitions that have been validated allows practitioners to be confident that the information they collect about families is accurate. Doing this also allows for systematic decision making about when to offer and conclude intervention. Data collected in this manner produce a clear picture of skills needed and skills learned. The data can be useful to show families the changes they have made or not made and to use in supervision. The data are based on fact, not supposition or intuition. If data cannot be collected in the manner we have suggested because of time or training constraints, we still strongly encourage the use of the protocols offered here in the systematic manner in which they have been designed and validated.

6

Home Safety and Cleanliness Training

Five percent of home accident fatalities involve children between birth and 4 years of age (National Safety Council, 2000). The causes of these fatalities include fire- or burn-related accidents, suffocation, drowning, falling, poisonings, and various other causes, such as firearms or electrocution. Of all reported incidences of child maltreatment, the majority involve physical neglect (U.S. Department of Health and Human Services, 1993). The presence of hazards in the homes of parents who have been reported for physical neglect may pose additional risks to children. When children are unsupervised, the risk of accidental death or injury may be greater.

The Home Accident Prevention Inventory—Revised (HAPI-R; see Tertinger et al., 1984, for original reference for the HAPI) is an assessment system that quantifies potential home safety hazards and that can be used to evaluate the effectiveness of home safety training. It has been used as an objective and comprehensive assessment of home safety conditions and was recently revised to apply to home environments in urban areas (Mandel, Bigelow, & Lutzker, 1998; Metchikian, Mink, Bigelow, Lutzker, & Doctor, 1999). The Checklist for Living Environments to Assess Neglect (CLEAN; Watson-Perczel et al., 1988) is a tool that can be used to assess the cleanliness of home conditions. Both of these assessment measures can be used concurrently to assess cleanliness and safety and to evaluate the effectiveness of a comprehensive training program.

MATERIALS

- *Home Safety and Cleanliness Assessment Participant Consent.* This consent form should be completed before beginning cleanliness and safety assessment. This form can be found in Appendix 6.1.
- *Family Session Summary.* As described in Chapter 3, this form lists tasks planned for each session. See Appendix 4.1.

- *Home Accident Prevention Inventory—Revised (HAPI-R) Data Sheet.* This is the sheet used to record the number of accessible hazards in families' homes. See Appendix 6.2.
- *Checklist for Living Environments to Assess Neglect (CLEAN) Data Sheet.* This is used to collect data on the cleanliness of families' homes. See Appendix 6.3.
- *Consumer Satisfaction Questionnaire.* Use this questionnaire to inquire about parent's satisfaction with the safety and cleanliness training program and its results. See Appendix 6.4.

INTRODUCING SAFETY AND CLEANLINESS ASSESSMENT

Because observations of home safety and cleanliness conditions involve looking around private areas of families' homes, it is important to discuss this process with the family beforehand and to obtain their consent to look through individual areas within their home. A consent form is included here as Appendix 6.1. A rationale for conducting the home safety observations should be provided to parents. This may include the following points:

"One area of interest is home safety."

"We would like to thoroughly evaluate how safe your home is for your children. To do so, the counselor would like to look through your home to find areas that pose potential risks to your children. We recognize that this may seem very invasive, but our main concern is making your home safe for you and your children."

"Allowing us to look through your home in the areas you have allowed us to look will help us provide specific information and assistance to make your home as safe as possible for you and your children."

You might explain that you will be looking through the home "from the child's-eye level" to find all of the hazards that children are likely to find. Reassure the parents that you will look only in areas for which they have given you permission to observe. The HAPI-R involves looking at any area that is accessible to the children in the home. These areas might include in drawers and cabinets, under beds, in closets, and in any containers that are accessible to children, such as jewelry boxes or nightstands. For this reason, parents are given the opportunity to state which areas in each room are off-limits. Before you begin home safety and cleanliness assessments, however, it is extremely important for you to have gained initial rapport and trust with families in order for them to feel comfortable allowing you access to private areas within their home. Often, if this is not accomplished, parents may decline participation in this component of the program; or they may initially consent to participate but feel uncomfortable or imposed on. Further, parents may withdraw from the program or not attend sessions in which safety and cleanliness observations are to be conducted. Although fostering a good working relationship with parents in which they are comfortable and fully engaged in the program is important at any time, it is especially important if counselors will be asking to look throughout the most private areas of a family's home. Counselors should keep in mind what it might be like to have service providers looking through every drawer and closet in their own homes. Throughout the assessment, counselors should be sure to leave all of the family's belongings in the same condition as before the assessment. For example, if the counselor needs to remove items from a drawer to count the number of accessible hazards, those items should be returned to the exact location at which they were originally found.

The next section provides definitions and instructions for conducting HAPI-R observations. Instructions for conducting CLEAN observations are in the following section. Then instructions for conducting home safety and cleanliness training are provided.

HOME ACCIDENT PREVENTION INVENTORY—REVISED

The HAPI-R is a relatively straightforward and simple measure of accessible hazards within a home. The number of hazards in eight major categories is counted. Within each category, individual hazards are listed, so that the frequency of each specific type of hazard can be determined. An HAPI-R score is obtained for each room in the home. Observations are conducted at each training session so that the number of accessible hazards within each room can be tracked over time.

Learning how to use the HAPI-R is an important step in conducting home safety training. This section contains definitions of accessibility and subcategories of hazards and observer instructions for conducting assessment sessions. An HAPI-R data sheet is included as Appendix 6.2.

Definitions

Definition of "Accessible"

Among the following conditions, either "1" or "2," in combination with either "3" or "4," must exist for a hazard to be scored as accessible.

1. A hazardous object (defined subsequently) is within arm's reach of any child, 0 to 6 years old, as he or she stands on the floor.
2. A hazardous object is within arm's reach of any child, 0 to 6-years-old, when he or she stands or climbs onto adjacent objects.
3. A hazardous object is in an open (unlocked) container or space.
4. A hazardous object does not have a childproof cap or lock or has a childproof cap or lock that is broken, cracked, or open.

Note: A child can climb onto any surface that is lower than his or her eye level. A child can step up or climb onto a series of progressively higher surfaces if they are arranged in a stair-step fashion and are lower than the child's eye level when the child is standing on each preceding surface level. Only record accessible stair-step surfaces that you encounter and measure during the time of your observation. Do not score surfaces as accessible under the assumption that a child could move an object, allowing him or her to step up to that surface.

For infants and children who are not yet walking, standard measures of 33 inches for eye level and 45 inches for reach may be used.

Categories and Definitions of Safety Hazards

The following eight general categories of hazards are defined.

1. Fire and electrical hazards
2. Hazardous ingestible small objects
3. Hazardous mechanical objects
4. Firearm hazards
5. Solid and liquid poisonous hazards
6. Hazardous sharp objects
7. Falling hazards
8. Drowning hazards

Within each of these categories are several subcategories of hazardous objects. When observing clients' homes, count the number of hazards encountered, following the "Observer Instructions" later in this chapter. Place slash marks in the appropriate boxes on the data sheet. Be sure to conduct separate observations for each room. Data for two rooms may be placed on one data sheet.

FIRE AND ELECTRICAL HAZARDS

This category of hazards includes combustibles, protective fire screens, electrical outlets and switches, protective appliance covers, and electrical cords and plugs. Accidents with these hazards can result in minor or severe burns, shocks, and/or death by electrocution.

Combustibles. Count the number of all accessible combustibles, defined as any substance that has the capability to create fire and/or explosions. These include matches, cigarette lighters, explosives, fireworks, ammunition, or fireplace additives. *Note: A box of matches, a book of matches, a box containing many packs of matches, or one match are all scored as one item.*

Protective fire screens. Count the number of fireplaces without a protective guard or screen. In addition, count the number of wood-burning stoves, furnaces, or space heaters without properly installed fire doors or protective screens. Include space heaters (portable and built-in) that have wire covers with spaces through which a child can put his or her hands.

Electrical outlets and switches. Count the number of electrical outlets and/or switches that have plates missing or improperly installed plates (that is, plates that do not come in contact with the wall surface, leaving a gap of more than ¼ inch, allowing for insertion of a child's fingertip). An "electrical outlet" is defined as an appropriate material covering for the receptacle that comes in contact with the wall surface. An "electrical switch plate" is defined as a device for turning electric currents on and off. A "switch plate" is defined as an appropriate material covering for the switch that touches the wall surface.

Protective Appliance Covers. Count the number of protective coverings placed on any operational electrical appliance (e.g., televisions sets, radios, computers, stereos, fans, blenders, etc.) by the manufacturer that are missing. *Note: An appliance is defined as "operational" if it is plugged into an electrical outlet. This may also include small appliances that are unplugged but used frequently. Ask a family member whether an unplugged appliance is used frequently. In addition, it is necessary to observe the side, back, and bottom of all accessible appliances.*

Electrical cords/plugs. Count the number of all damaged appliance and extension cords and plugs, that is, any cord that is cracked, frayed, and/or showing exposed wires and any plug with missing pans. Cords or plugs that have been appropriately repaired or securely wrapped with electrical tape are excluded from the count. *Note: Stereo speaker wires, cable TV wires, and telephone wires are also excluded because they carry low electric currents that will not result in shocks. However, the wires from stereo components (for example, amplifier, turntable) do carry high electric currents and should be observed for damage.*

HAZARDOUS INGESTIBLE SMALL OBJECTS

This category of hazards includes ingestible small objects. Accidents with small objects can result in suffocation by obstruction of the throat or in internal damage or in poisoning by ingestion.

Ingestible Small Objects. Count the number of any small objects accessible to an infant or young child (i.e., on the floor, on low furniture, in playpens and cribs, etc.). To determine if an item is considered a "small object," insert the object into a no-choke measuring tube or an empty toilet paper roll (measuring 1 ⅝ inches in diameter). If the object falls completely into the tube or the toilet paper roll, it fails the U.S. Consumer Product Safety Commission Test and may result in airway obstruction or ingestion by young children (especially children under the age of 3). If any part of the object sticks out of the tube, then it is not considered a "small ingestible object." *Note: If small objects are consolidated and found in a jar or other container, all small objects are scored as one* hazard and not counted separately. A "container" is defined as any object that will hold the small objects in place. It should have sides that would sufficiently keep the small objects in place when tilted. In addition to common small ingestible objects, such as small toys, uncooked beans and pasta, staples, small magnets placed on a refrigerator, potpourri, and any other accessible object that would fit in the No-Choke tube should be recorded as hazards. If an item could be categorized as "small" and "sharp," such as pins, needles, or staples, categorize that item as "small."

HAZARDOUS MECHANICAL OBJECTS

This category of hazards includes crib cords and plastics. Accidents with these hazards can result in strangulation or suffocation by mechanical means. Parents often dangle toys and colorful objects across cribs, playpens, or other play areas using cords or ropes. Small infants may pull themselves up onto the cords and fall with the cord pressing into the throat, resulting in accidental strangulation. In addition, young children will often be fascinated by sheets of flexible plastic and place them over their mouths and noses, resulting in suffocation.

Crib Cords. Count the number of cords accessible to infants (e.g., in cribs, playpens, or designated sleeping or play areas). A "cord" is defined as a string or small rope consisting of several woven strands of rope, string, plastics, wires, and so forth. Include hanging telephone or appliance cords if they are easily accessible to children. This does not include cords that are thick and unlikely to loop around a child's neck, cords that lie on the floor, or cords that are behind furniture or otherwise inaccessible. *Note: Score this category only if the family actually uses a crib, playpen, or other designated areas for containing a child during sleep or play periods. It may be necessary to determine "designated areas" by asking your client.*

Plastics. Count the number of accessible plastic bags and thin plastic materials. Garbage bags lining waste containers and other plastic items (for example, cellophane wraps or bags) stored in an original container are excluded from the count. In addition, plastic bags containing items for storage are not counted. If several plastic bags, such as grocery bags, are stored in one plastic bag, then count all of the plastics stored in that one bag as one. *Note: A plastic is considered a hazard if it is large enough to cover both the mouth and nose at the same time. For example, a soft, disposable plastic glove is a hazard, but a plastic glove of the type used for dishwashing is not because it is thick and unlikely to adhere to a child's nose and mouth.*

FIREARM HAZARDS

This category of hazards includes all firearms that may result in accidental shootings. Children are often interested in guns. If accessible and handled incorrectly, a shooting can result in severe physical damage or death.

Firearms. Count the number of all accessible firearms (i.e., guns, rifles, BB pistols, air-pump BB guns, machine guns, etc.). *Do not handle any firearm to determine if it is loaded or locked. Score all accessible firearms.*

SOLID AND LIQUID POISONOUS HAZARDS

This category contains many hazards, including pill medications, tube medications, inhaler medications, liquid medications, jar medications, alcoholic beverages, beauty products, detergents and cleansers, deodorizers, polishes and waxes, paints and stains, solvents and thinners, glues and adhesives, poisonous plants, herbicides and fertilizers, insecticides and rodenticides, and petroleum products. Accidents can result in illness, poisoning, burns, abrasions, and rashes. If a child swallows a solid or liquid poison, severe illness, poisoning, or internal damage could result. In addition, if a child mishandles solid or liquid hazards, chemical burns, rashes, abrasions, or blindness could result.

Pill Medications. Count the number of all accessible, nonchildproof pill containers, defined as a bottle or box containing pill, capsule, or tablet medications. These include medications that are wrapped in foil, paper, or plastic (e.g., suppositories, throat lozenges) and vitamins. A "childproof container" is defined as a container that a child cannot open (for example, prescription containers with caps that require more than a simple turn to open). The childproof container must be properly closed or sealed.

Tube Medications. Count the number of all accessible tube medications, defined as any medication contained in a small collapsible cylinder of metal or plastic that has one sealed end and a capped opening from which the medication is applied. Toothpaste and empty tubes are excluded from this count.

Inhaler Medications. Count the number of all accessible inhaler medications, that is, those contained in cylindrical-shaped devices usually made of plastic that are used to administer inhaled medicinal vapors. Bottled liquid medications are excluded from this count.

Liquid Medications. Count the number of accessible, nonchildproofed liquid medications, that is, any container of medicinal fluid. These include droppers, eyedrops, sprays, and aerosols (for example, mouthwash, antibacterial spray, hydrogen peroxide, iodine, rubbing alcohol, cough medicine).

Jar Medications. Count the number of accessible jar medications, that is, those in broadmouthed, usually cylindrical glass or plastic containers that hold gelled medication (for example, Vicks VapoRub or Vaseline—note that petroleum jellies are scored under *this category* rather than as petroleum products, listed later).

Alcoholic Beverages. Count the number of accessible alcoholic beverages, defined as any ingestible distilled fruit or grain spirit. These include "hard" alcohol, wine, wine coolers, beer, liquors, champagnes, cordials, and so forth. *Note: An intact 6-pack, 12-pack, or case of beer or wine coolers is scored as one hazard even if the pack is opened.*

Beauty Products. Count the number of accessible beauty products, defined as any item used for facial or body cosmetic purposes. These include fingernail polish remover, cologne, perfume, toilet water, deodorant, eye makeup, hair bleach, hair dye, hair neutralizer, hair rinse, hair setting, hair spray, hair straightener, hair tint, hair tonic, facial makeup, permanent wave solution, astringent, lotions, bath oil, cosmetic creams, shaving lotions, skin creams, suntan preparations, lipstick, shampoo, conditioner, bath powder, bath salts, bleach cream, cuticle cream, cuticle remover, hair remover products, shaving powder, feminine deodorants, lip balm, contact lens preparations, baby products (e.g., shampoos, lotions, powders), and bubble bath. This *excludes toothpaste and tooth powders.*

Detergents and Cleansers. Count the number of accessible detergents and cleansers, defined as any substance used for cleaning household surfaces or areas. These include powders, sprays, liquids, aerosols, fabric treatment agents, tablet cleansers, soap pads, degreasers, rug shampoo, bleaches, softeners, fabric softeners, shoe preparations, auto cleansers, and jewelry cleanser. This *excludes bars of facial or bath soaps and liquid hand soap.*

Deodorizers. Count the number of accessible deodorizers, defined as any substance that is used for removing unwanted smells from living spaces or items. These include solid, spray, car, diaper pail, and wardrobe deodorizers. *Note: This also includes solid deodorizers hanging in toilet bowls that are considered accessible but excludes solid deodorizers hanging in inaccessible toilet tanks.*

Polishes and Waxes. Count the number of accessible polishes and waxes, defined as any substance used to polish, wax, or oil a household surface or personal clothing items (for example, shoe polish). These include pastes, polishes, waxes, sprays, and/or oils used on wooden, floor, furniture, appliance, auto, or leather surfaces. In addition, "no-wax" furniture polishes are included in this count.

Paints and Stains. Count the number of accessible paints and stains, defined as any substance used to preserve, treat, or seal household surfaces or used in an artistic fashion. *Note: Score all accessible paint cans, stain cans, and spray paints even if the lids are tightly fitted.*

Solvents and Thinners. Count the number of accessible solvents and thinners, defined as any chemical substance used to dissolve or thin another substance. These include paint thinners, stain removers, paint strippers, antifreeze, windshield wiper fluid, deicers, record, tape, and CD head cleaners, correction fluid for paper, and alcohol-based dry cleaning fluid.

Glues and Adhesives. Count the number of accessible glues and adhesives, defined as any substance used to bond two surfaces together. This includes glues, cohesives, and adhesives (for example, household glue, auto seal, glass seal, patching plaster, caulking, carpet adhesive, rubber cement). This *excludes tapes and glues that are labeled as nontoxic.*

Poisonous Plants. Count the number of accessible toxic plants. The following common household plants are poisonous: oleander, dieffenbachia (dumb cane), narcissus, caladium, hyacinths, solanum (Christmas cherry), and mistletoe. The following descriptions identify these plants; illustrations of the plants may be found in common gardening books.

1. *Oleander.* Oleander is a tall shrub with lance-shaped leaves that are leathery, sharp-pointed, and appear in whorls of three. Fruits are long and slender and seeds are hairy. Oleanders are commonly used as ornamental potted plants.

- *Toxic parts.* Entire plant, especially the leaves. A single leaf can kill an adult or child who chews or sucks on the leaf. Inhaling the smoke from burned branches or eating food that has been cooked using the branches as a skewer can result in severe poisoning.
- *Symptoms.* Nausea, severe vomiting, stomach pain, bloody diarrhea, dizziness, slowed pulse, cold extremities, irregular heartbeat, dilated pupils, drowsiness, unconsciousness, paralysis of the lungs, convulsions, coma, and death, usually within 24 hours.

2. *Dieffenbachia (dumb cane).* Dumb canes are tall shrubby plants that can reach 6 feet in height. The leaves are large, oblong, and entirely green or mottled white and green. Plants have a skunk-like odor when bruised. Dumb canes are very common ornamentals.

- *Toxic parts*. Entire plants, especially the stems. If eaten or chewed, severe burning and swelling occurs in the throat and mouth. The swelling may interfere with speech, swallowing, and breathing for 1 week or more. In severe cases, swollen tongues and mouths can result in death by choking; however, deaths have not been reported in humans.
- *Symptoms*. Severe burning and swelling of the mucous membranes of the mouth and throat, choking, nausea, vomiting, diarrhea, and copious salivation.

3. *Narcissus*. Narcissus is a spring-flowering bulbous herb with long, narrow leaves with parallel veins. White or yellow flowers occur four to eight on a stalk. Narcissus may be grown indoors or outdoors.

- *Toxic parts*. Bulbs. Eating even a small amount of the bulb may cause poisoning. The plants may also cause contact dermatitis in sensitive individuals.
- *Symptoms*. Severe digestive upset, including nausea, vomiting, and diarrhea, trembling, minor convulsions, and in some cases, death.

4. *Caladium*. Caladium is a stemless plant with large, varicolored heart-shaped leaves and tuberous roots. Caladium is a common houseplant.

- *Toxic parts*. All parts, especially the leaves and tubers. Chewed or eaten parts will result in tissue paralysis, burning, and swelling.
- *Symptoms*. Severe burning of the mouth and throat, swelling of the tongue and throat, choking, nausea, vomiting, diarrhea, and salivation. Death may occur if tissues in the back of the tongue swell enough to block breathing.

5. *Hyacinths*. Hyacinths are bulbous herbs with long, narrow leaves. Flowers are white, yellow, pink, red, or blue in a cluster at the end of the stalk. Plants are commonly grown in pots and gardens.

- *Toxic parts*. Bulbs. Eating a small amount of the bulbs may cause poisoning. The plants may also cause contact dermatitis in sensitive individuals.
- *Symptoms*. Intense stomach cramps, nausea, vomiting, and diarrhea.

6. *Solanum (Christmas cherry)*. The Christmas or Jerusalem cherry is a smooth erect shrub with oblong, pointed, glossy, and wavy leaves. Flowers are white and fruits are round berries, either bright red or orange. The plants are typically shown at Christmas time for their showy berries.

- *Toxic parts*. Entire plant, especially the leaves and unripened berries. Unripened berries are extremely toxic, and small amounts can be deadly. However, severe poisoning is rare, because most cases result from eating the relatively nontoxic ripe berries.

- *Symptoms*. Headache, stomach pain, subnormal temperature, vomiting, diarrhea, convulsions, respiratory and central nervous system depression, paralysis, dilated pupils, and loss of sensation. In severe cases, death can result.

7. *Mistletoe*. Mistletoe may have green or white, oblong; leathery leaves. Flowers are small and usually embedded in a stalk. Fruits are small white berries. Mistletoe is a commonly displayed ornamental during the Christmas season.

- *Toxic parts*. All parts, especially the berries. Persons can be poisoned by eating or making tea with the berries.
- *Symptoms*. Nausea, vomiting, nervousness, difficulty breathing, delirium, hallucinations, dilation of the pupils, miscarriage, convulsions, heart failure, stomach and intestinal pains, diarrhea, slow pulse, and collapse. Death may occur within a few hours.

Herbicides and Fertilizers. Count the number of accessible herbicides and fertilizers, defined as any substance used in the upkeep of household or garden plants. These include herbicides, fertilizers, and plant food.

Insecticides and Rodenticides. Count the number of accessible insecticides and rodenticides, defined as any substance used to repel, deter, or poison insects and/or animals. These include insect repellents, small and large animal repellents, flea dips and shampoos, flea collars (do not count collars on pets), fly strips, mothballs, rat poison, and insecticide towelettes.

Petroleum Products. Count the number of accessible petroleum products, defined as any substance made with a petroleum base that may be flammable. These include gasoline, kerosene, lighter fluids, charcoal products, and lubricants.

HAZARDOUS SHARP OBJECTS

This category of hazards includes sharp objects that may result in minor or severe cuts, abrasions, or punctures.

Sharp Objects. Count the number of accessible sharp objects, defined as any item with sharpened edges or points that could cause a laceration or puncture wound. These include knives, forks, scissors, ice picks, corkscrews, awls, nails, screws, hooks, fireplace pokers, skewers, and so forth. This category also includes broken glass or hard plastic items. Items such as pencils and pens are *not* included in the count. *Note: If several sharp objects are consolidated in one cabinet or drawer (e.g., ten sharp knives and a pair of scissors) without being in a single container, as in a silverware tray, count the items individually. If the items are in a container inside a drawer or cabinet (silverware trays are included as containers), then count the items as only one. If an item could be categorized as "small" and "sharp," such as pins, needles, or staples, categorize that item as "small."*

FALLING HAZARDS

This category of hazards includes balconies, steps, and windows, which may result in accidental falls, severe injury or death.

Balconies. Count the number of balconies accessible to children. Accessibility is defined as the absence of doors, safety locks, bars, or other devices that prevent children from going onto the balcony without supervision.

Steps. Count the number of accessible stairways or sets of steps. These are defined as any stairway or set of steps that does not have a gate or other device at the bottom and top to prevent an infant's access to it. Stairways should have a banister on at least one side, with bars spaced close enough so that a child's head cannot become stuck in between them. *Note: Score each missing gate or safety device as one hazard, so that a stairway missing a gate at both the top and the bottom is scored as two hazards. Score a missing banister as one hazard and a banister with widely spaced bars (that is, so that a child's head can become stuck) as one hazard.*

Windows. Count the number of accessible windows, defined as any window that the child can reach that is large enough for a child to fit through (approximately 8–10 inches) and that does not have a safety lock, securely attached screen, or bars to prevent the child from climbing or falling through it. *Note: Bars must be spaced close enough together so that the child's head cannot get stuck between them; if not, score as one hazard. In addition, a window without a safety device is scored as a hazard only if the child can reach it, such as by climbing on furniture beneath or beside it.*

DROWNING HAZARDS

This category of hazards includes bathtubs and sinks, buckets, and wading pools that pose the risk of accidental drowning.

Bathtubs/sinks. Count the number of accessible bathtubs or sinks that contain water or other liquids.

Buckets. Count the number of accessible buckets and other open containers that contain non-poisonous liquid, such as water. *Note: Poisonous liquids (for example, cleaning detergents) should be counted as a hazard under the category of solid and liquid poisonous hazards.*

Wading Pools. Count the number of wading pools accessible to children. A wading pool is considered accessible if it has water in it and if the child can get to it without adult supervision.

Note: Liquid that is at least half an inch deep should be recorded as a hazard. Infants can drown from inhaling water, not only from becoming immersed in liquid.

Observer Instructions

I. Preparation and data collection
    A. Before you begin an HAPI-R assessment, you need to secure your client's signature on an informed consent form. A copy of a sample consent form is given as Appendix 6.1. The consent form should be read over thoroughly before beginning assessment. Any of the parents' questions or concerns should be addressed, and parents' restrictions on areas that may be observed should be honored.
    B. To conduct an HAPI-R assessment, you will need a copy of the HAPI-R assessment manual for reference, data sheets, a tape measure, a no-choke test tube, pen or pencil, and a clipboard.
    C. Write the following information on the HAPI-R data sheet:
        1. Client's name
        2. Date of assessment
        3. Observer's name
        4. Measurement of the largest child's eye level and reach
        5. Rooms being assessed in the home (do not list more than two rooms per data sheet)
II. Measurement of child accessibility
    A. Identify the physically largest child between the ages of 0 and 6 years.
    B. Measure the child from eye level to the floor when the child is standing up straight and feet are placed together.
    C. With the child standing up straight, feet placed together, arm outstretched directly overhead, measure the child from the tip of the hand to the floor.
    D. If the oldest children in the home are infants and are not walking, use standard measures of 33 inches for eye level and 45 inches for reach.
    E. Record the measurements on the data sheet so they are available for your use when assessing the home for hazards. Use these measurements when assessing the accessibility of higher surfaces (for example, counter- and tabletops, shelves, cabinets, etc.) Remember, if a surface is at the eye level of a child, he or she can climb onto that surface.
III. Record the number of hazards for each subcategory in the space provided for each room. Systematically assess each room by walking around and observing the room in a clockwise fashion. You should observe the room only one time. As you identify hazards, place a tally mark in the appropriate space for each subcategory. After completing each room, add the tally marks for each subcategory of hazards.
IV. General rules when conducting HAPI-R assessments
    A. Complete the assessment one room at a time.
    B. Keep the measuring tape with you throughout data collection. It may be convenient to drape the tape measure loosely around your neck.
    C. Open cabinets to see if shelves can be used by the child as steps. Shelves may serve as steps, thus changing the accessibility of other nearby objects. *Note: Do not open cabinets and other closed areas if your client has not given you consent.*

D. If a drawer, cabinet, shelf, dresser, or countertop is within arm's reach of the child, count all accessible hazards in the drawer or cabinet or on the shelf or countertop. A drawer, cabinet, shelf, dresser, or countertop are within arm's reach if the child can touch the following locations:
    1. If the child can touch any portion of the bottom inside surface of the drawer, then all items in that drawer are accessible.
    2. If the child can touch any portion of its top surface, then all items on top of the cabinet, shelf, dresser, or countertop are accessible.
E. If a sink can be used for climbing to other nearby locations, determine further accessible areas by measuring from the bowl of the sink.
F. If there is a question regarding the contents of a container, ask the parent.
G. The definition of "childproof" caps with locks may also include containers that have directions written on them (for example, "Squeeze the arrows on the cap to open"). Remember to check all containers for childproof packaging, not just medications. By way of example, some insecticides have childproof packaging. Further, check to be sure that all caps with locks are actually secured and not just placed on top of the container such that the childproof mechanisms are not in effect.
H. When assessing hazards that are considered a "set," such as a box containing a set of oil paints or a set of contact lens preparations, count the set as one hazard. A good guideline when trying to determine if something is a set is to determine whether the objects are related or used for the same general purpose. In addition, score hazards that are consolidated in a container as one item.
I. Occasionally, hazardous objects can be scored under more than one category. When this occurs, score the item under the most appropriate category using your best judgment—do not score the hazard twice. The most common example is small objects that are sharp (such as a package of tacks or small nails.). In these cases score the hazard under "Small Objects" rather than "Sharp Objects."
J. The HAPI-R does not directly quantify some hazardous substances, including garbage and spoiling food. Make a note of whether your client has open garbage (that is, garbage that is not contained or contained without an appropriate cover) or spoiling food at the bottom of the data sheet. Do not forget to check your client's garbage container and refrigerator.

CHECKLIST FOR LIVING ENVIRONMENTS TO ASSESS NEGLECT (CLEAN)

Having a clean home environment is an important part of having a safe home. A messy or dirty home environment can also interfere with other clinical treatment goals. For example, it may not be feasible to conduct PCI skills training when the home is so dirty that a child's health is at risk. Therefore, a family's goals often include improving the home's physical condition to reduce health hazards and increase safety. The following are procedures for assessing the cleanliness of a home. These procedures can be used with the Home Accident Prevention Inventory—Revised Data Sheet or independent of this assessment.

When using the CLEAN, "item areas" (for example, furniture, surface areas, fixtures, appliances) are inspected. The resulting data are transformed into a "composite percentage score" ranging from 0 to 100%, with higher scores indicating higher overall cleanliness conditions. A more detailed description of the CLEAN is given in the following.

The CLEAN measures three dimensions that contribute to the overall cleanliness condition of a home. These dimensions are (1) Clean/Dirty, (2) Clothes/Linens Not Belonging, and (3) Number of Objects Not Belonging. The following definitions describe how these dimensions are quantified and scored using the CLEAN.

Dimension of Cleanliness Definitions

Clean/Dirty

An area is scored "Dirty" only if one or more of the following conditions exist:

1. There is more than one square inch of continuous *Organic decaying matter (ODM)* in direct contact with the item area. ODM includes any organic matter that is decaying or has potential for supporting fungus, algae, mold, or insect larvae. Examples include spilled human or pet food, grease spots, heavy dust, food liquids, crumbs, dead insects, and so forth.
2. There is more than one square inch of continuous *nonorganic matter (NOM)* in direct contact with the item area. NOM includes any nonorganic matter such as spilled liquid chemicals, petroleum products, cosmetic material, and so forth.

Clothes/Linens (CLs)

Each CL resting on or in an item area that does not belong there is counted.

1. A clothing item is defined as any article that is worn by a person, including shirts, blouses, pants, skirts, coats, shoes, hats, socks, gloves, scarves, and so forth.
2. A linen item is any cloth or material article other than clothing, including towels, sheets, tablecloths, handkerchiefs, and so forth.

Objects Not Belonging (NBs)

Each NB that is determined as not belonging on or in a specific item area is counted. An NB is defined as any object that can be thrown away or that has a more specific, appropriate storage place other than the item area in observation. NBs include used dishes (outside of the kitchen sink), open or spoiled perishable foods not in direct contact with an item area, garbage, hazardous items, toys, cosmetics (outside of the bathroom), tools, purses, pocketbooks, wallets, old papers, tissues or paper towels, doll clothing, and so forth.

CLEAN Scoring Rules

In addition to the CLEAN dimension definitions, there are scoring rules for observing specific characteristics of each household room:

Kitchen
- Dirty dishes in sink are not scored unless piled above the counter level. All dishes, pans, pots, and so forth above the counter level are counted individually as NBs.
- Dishes that are clean and left out to air dry in the sink, on the counter, or in a drying rack are excluded from the NB count.
- Splashed water around the sink is not an indication of "Dirty" unless the water contains ODM.
- If data collection occurs during regular mealtimes, dishes and utensils on the table, stove, and sink are excluded from the NB count. In addition, fresh cooking or eating spills are not an indication of "Dirty."
- One washcloth and two towels (for a minimum of three) hung to dry are excluded from the CL count.
- Bread and fruit stored on kitchen counters are excluded from the NB count. Bread must be in a bag or other container and fruit must be unused.

Living room
- Two toys per child on the floor are excluded from the NB count. In addition, if a child has a set-up consolidated play area with many toy items (e.g., battlefield, train set, or "Barbie Neighborhood") that is used regularly, it is excluded from the NB count.

Bathroom
- A cup or tumbler on or near the sink is excluded from the NB count.
- Cosmetic products used daily are allowable if they are not hazardous and are stored appropriately (for example, placed in a drawer or on shelves versus stored in the sink).
- One washcloth and/or towel per person hung to dry are excluded from the CL count.

Bedroom
- Two toys per child on the floor of children's bedrooms are excluded from the NB count. In addition, if a child has a set-up consolidated play area with many toy items (similar to the examples used for the living room) that is used regularly, it is excluded from the NB count.

Miscellaneous
- Stains are an indication of "Dirty" furniture, floor carpets, sheets, counters, and so forth. Touch any stain to determine whether it is permanent or removable. Permanent stains that have been cleaned are not an indicator of "Dirty."
- A consolidated pile of papers or other very small objects is scored as one NB.
- A consolidated box of paper of other objects is scored as one NB.
- A pile of feces makes an item area "Dirty" but is not counted as an NB.

- A very thin layer of dust is not an indication of "Dirty." Score dusty item areas as "Dirty" only when the dust is thick enough to ball up.
- NBs are sometimes difficult to determine. If a particular object is in question, ask your client where they typically store that item. If you are still unsure about the "appropriateness" of the storage area, use the following guidelines to determine if an object is an NB:

    1. Safety: If the item is hazardous and within a child's reach, it should be scored as an NB without exception.
    2. Function: If an item area has a certain function, then objects related to that function are not scored as NBs (e.g., eyeglasses placed on a "reading table," salt and pepper shakers on a dining room table, a stack of magazines neatly stored on a coffee table).

Observer Instructions and Data Collection Procedure

Identifying Item Areas

Each room of the home requires the use of a separate data sheet for every session. First determine if only outer surfaces of item areas will be observed or if interiors of item areas (that is, inside closets, drawers, etc.) will be included in the observation. If an HAPI-R is also being conducted, that assessment will account for hazards inside of drawers or closets, so it may not be necessary or practical to also require the inside of these areas to meet the CLEAN guidelines.

Before you collect CLEAN data, you will need to generate a list of "item areas" for each room. Use the following guidelines when defining item areas:

1. An item area can be defined as any item and/or area that has discrete and observable boundaries, including chairs, tables, sinks, bathtubs, toilets, countertops, furniture, walls, floor, closets, oven, inside the refrigerator, and so forth.
2. All rooms should include the walls and floor as item areas. Certain areas with large surface areas (e.g., countertops or floors) should be broken into several areas by using naturally occurring boundaries (e.g., a couch dividing a living room into two halves). In addition, homes often have several item areas that are similar (for example, two large chairs). When this occurs, label the areas with descriptive terms so that new observers can identify the appropriate item area. Some examples include "Stove Counter," "North Sink," "Floor behind Couch," "Flowered Chair," or "Recliner."

Scoring a Room

Item areas should be listed along the left-hand column of the CLEAN data sheet. After defining item areas for each room, follow the procedure below for data collection:

1. Fill out the information required at the top of every data sheet *including your name, the date of observation, and client's name, the room, and the session number.* Also, circle Bl—baseline, or pretraining sessions; T—training sessions; or F—follow-up sessions.
2. As you enter each room, make a subjective rating concerning the room's overall appearance. At the top right corner of each data sheet indicate whether the room's over-

all appearance is good (+), very poor (–), or neither good nor bad (0) by circling the appropriate symbol.

3. Begin observations at the first item area listed on the data sheet. For each item area, determine the following:

   - Whether the item area is Clean or Dirty. Place a check mark in the appropriate box on the data sheet.
   - Moving across the data sheet to the right, count the number of Clothes/Linens. Count all the CLs and check the appropriate number range on the data sheet.
   - Count the number of Objects Not Belonging. Check the appropriate number range on the data sheet.

4. Repeat the procedure until all item areas are scored in all rooms.

5. At the bottom of each data sheet is space for comments. Indicate any information that may be important for that data collection session for treatment purposes. For example, there might be an unusually large number of roaches or spiders present; however, the CLEAN does not measure insects, and the information might be important. In addition, for the kitchen and bathrooms, note the presence or absence of a minimum of cleaning supplies and garbage containers.

6. After each data collection trial, summarize your data using the instructions at the bottom of the data sheet. Four percentage scores can be obtained from CLEAN data:

   - The *Composite Cleanliness Percentage Score* yields a composite score that summarizes the whole room's condition. To calculate the composite score, first summarize each "item area score" by adding the appropriate point values for Clean/Dirty, CLs, and NBs. Place the totals in the right-hand column and add. Place this total in the "total ratings" space. Next, count the number of item areas and enter the total. Divide the total of item area scores by the number of item areas, then divide the resulting quotient by 20. Last, multiply the quotient by 100 to yield the Composite Cleanliness Percentage Score. Following the instructions on the CLEAN data sheet will give you this score.
   - A *Percentage of Clean Item Areas* is calculated simply by adding the number of clean item areas and dividing by the total number of item areas. Multiply the quotient by 100 to yield the percentage. Use the "total points" spaces provided at the bottom of the data sheet for summarizing this information. If an initial score is greater than 80%, no additional assessments or training on home cleanliness need take place unless you observe the home to become cluttered or dirty throughout the remainder of your contact.
   - The last two percentage scores use the bottom "total" boxes in order to calculate the *Percentage of Points Earned for CLs* and *Percentage of Points Earned for NBs*. These are calculated by adding the number of points earned for each item area and writing those scores in the "total points" boxes along the bottom of each column. Each score can then be divided by the total possible number of points for all item areas in a given dimension (CL or NB). Then multiply the quotient by 100 to yield the *Percentage of Points Earned*.

HOME SAFETY AND CLEANLINESS TRAINING PROTOCOL

Home safety training is provided to families in order to improve the conditions of families' homes, thus making the homes safer for children. In a safe home, hazards are inaccessible to young children. Hazards may be made inaccessible by one of three methods:

1. Using childproof latches
2. Using locks
3. Placing hazardous items out of the reach of children

Note: An item is out of a child's reach if the child cannot reach that item when standing on the floor or after climbing onto nearby furniture that is placed so that the surfaces can be used in a stair-step fashion. A child can climb onto furniture or other objects if the top of that object is at or below a child's eye level. By measuring the height of the oldest child's eye level and reach, we can determine whether items are accessible.

In Project SafeCare, many homes were observed to be clean and well kept, although many hazards were still present. In these cases, only home safety training was provided. If cleanliness appeared to be a problem, a CLEAN observation was conducted. If the initial CLEAN score was greater than 80%, the counselors did not conduct additional observations or provide cleanliness training unless a particular problem arose during the course of training.

The following protocol includes steps for conducting home safety and cleanliness training, but they may be modified to suit the needs of individual families. For instance, a home that is consistently neat and clean may still present risks to children. Each training session follows generally the same format. Training begins in one room of the house, and all safety hazards are targeted for that room. Subsequent training sessions identify safety hazards in other rooms. All hazards should be removed in the first room targeted for training before training in subsequent rooms begins. All hazards in the second room should be removed before training is conducted in the third room, and so on.

During each session, it is preferable to remove all hazards in the room, but if this is not feasible, parents should be asked to remove or make safe any remaining hazards before the next training session. A HAPI-R observation should be conducted in each room to ensure that previously trained rooms are hazard free and to determine which hazards still remain in rooms in which training is yet to be conducted.

Materials

For each training session, you will need to have the following materials:

- HAPI-R data sheets
- CLEAN data sheets
- Pencil
- Tape measure
- No-Choke tube

- Safety devices (as needed)
- Cleaning supplies (as needed)
- Screwdriver (if necessary for assisting with installation of child safety latches)

In Project SafeCare, parents were provided with outlet plugs and cabinet and drawer safety latches. If you will not be providing these to parents, they should be advised to obtain these items and to have several on hand at each training session.

Table 6.1 provides a concise overview of the session formats that are detailed in the following pages.

Session 1

The first session will probably be the longest because all home safety items and cleaning and safety strategies will be introduced. Subsequent sessions will probably take less time and will consist of reviewing the home safety items and applying safety strategies to different hazards in other rooms.

TABLE 6.1. Home Safety and Cleanliness Training Sessions

Session 1

   I. Pretraining observation
  II. Rationale for and description of training
 III. Establish the training agenda
  IV. Introduce cleanliness training
   V. Introduce safety training
  VI. Begin locating areas in need of cleaning and removing hazards
 VII. End the session

Sessions 2–4

   I. HAPI-R and CLEAN observation
  II. Review previous session's materials
 III. Review parent's hazard removal and cleaning since previous session and provide positive feedback for corrections made
  IV. Begin locating areas in need of cleaning and removing hazards
   V. End the session

Session 5

   I. HAPI-R and CLEAN observation
  II. Review of previous sessions materials
 III. Highlight important changes parent has made in home
  IV. Remind parent there is no substitute for parental supervision
   V. Problem solve strategies for clean, safe home
  VI. Anticipate future needed changes
 VII. Give positive feedback
VIII. Give parent a Consumer Satisfaction Questionnaire

I. Conduct a pretraining observation (HAPI-R and CLEAN) for each room (living room, kitchen, bedroom, bathroom, etc.). Do not provide any feedback or instruction yet.

II. Provide the rationale for and description of the training. Include the following points:
   A. Parents will learn to "childproof" their home to prevent serious accidents.
   B. Parents will learn to make the home a healthier and thus a safer place for a child.
   C. Training will take place over several visits in each of the home's rooms.
   D. Training will involve looking throughout the house for hazards and for areas to be cleaned.

III. Establish the training agenda.
   A. Instruction will focus on one room at a time. Identify the room in which training will begin (for example, the living room).
   B. Tell the parent that you will begin training by reviewing the health and safety hazards in the first room and that the parent will then have the opportunity to reduce and remove the target hazards in that room before training begins in the second room.
   C. During each training session, you will discuss and practice a variety of ways to make homes safe and clean for children.

IV. Introduce cleanliness training.
   A. Describe the three dimensions of cleanliness (refer to preceding definitions) and use examples from the target room to illustrate:
      1. Clean/dirty
      2. Clothes and linens not belonging
      3. Other objects not belonging
   B. Solicit and answer questions from the parent.
   C. Ask the parent to restate the dimensions of cleanliness.
   D. Discuss with the parent general methods for cleaning (that is, dusting, wiping with soap and water, vacuuming, sweeping and mopping, washing dishes, picking up items, cleaning spills, etc.).
   E. Ask parent to show you his or her cleaning supplies (cleansers, paper towels, broom, mop, etc.).

V. Introduce safety training
   A. Describe three ways to make hazards inaccessible:
      1. Use child-resistant closures.
      2. Lock up items.
      3. Place items out of child's reach.
   B. Solicit and answer questions from the parent.
   C. Ask the parent to restate the ways to make hazards inaccessible
   D. Describe how to determine if hazards are accessible.
      1. Children can reach anything they can touch while standing up straight with their arms held up above their heads.
      2. Children can climb onto any surface that is at or below their eye level. They can then climb up onto other higher surfaces, so it is necessary to ensure that these areas are safe and do not contain hazards.

      E. Solicit and answer questions from the parent.

      F. Ask the parent to restate the two ways in which areas within their home might be accessible to their children.

  VI. Begin locating areas in need of cleaning and removing hazards.

      A. Determine the room in which training will be conducted (based on which room poses the greatest hazards) and discuss with the parent whether it is a good day for working in that particular room.

      B. Give specific feedback about CLEAN score in this room.
         1. Identify one item area.
         2. Review definitions for dimensions of cleanliness and provide specific feedback and instructions for that area.

      C. Help parent clean the item area.
         1. Discuss methods to improve cleanliness of the area.
         2. Model methods if necessary.
         3. Identify other item areas and provide specific feedback.
         4. Give parent assignment to complete remaining item areas before next session.

      D. Provide feedback.
         1. Verbal, descriptive praise (for example, "Great, you organized all of the papers that were on this table.")
         2. Suggestions (for example, "In order to clean that area, you might neatly fold and stack the clothes.")

      E. Give specific feedback about HAPI score for that room (that is, "There are 15 hazards that I have found in this room, and we will begin to remove each of these hazards today").
         1. Describe the eight categories of hazards and how these hazards could endanger the lives of small children (refer to the HAPI-R assessment definitions given earlier in this chapter).
         2. Identify specific subcategories of hazards that are present in the current room.
         3. Review the three methods to make hazards inaccessible.

      F. Help the parent locate one hazard and demonstrate how it could be made inaccessible by one of the three methods.
         1. Describe the hazard and different strategies for making it inaccessible.
         2. When necessary, demonstrate how to use childproof devices such as drawer latches or cabinet locks.

      G. Have parent practice identifying and removing remaining hazards.
         1. Ask parent to locate a similar item (if she or he cannot, locate one for her or him)
         2. Ask parent to make hazard inaccessible.
         3. Provide feedback:
            a. Verbal, descriptive praise (e.g., "Good, you have placed the matches way up high and out of your child's reach").
            b. Suggestions (e.g., "In order to make that item inaccessible, you will need to put it in a place where there is no furniture a child can climb on to reach it").

      H. Continue to locate *all* hazardous items throughout the room.
         1. Model strategies for making items inaccessible.

2. Ask the parent to practice these strategies until all hazards have been identified and addressed.

3. Continue to provide feedback.

VII. *End the session.*

A. At the end of the session, review any hazards that remain.

B. Ask the parent to correct all hazards. If necessary, leave a checklist of specific hazards or areas to remind parents of the hazard and how it can be made inaccessible. With some families, it may be necessary to devise more creative strategies to prompt them to remove hazards and to continue to ensure that each room is safe. These strategies might include individualized checklists or charts or the use of Polaroid photographs to highlight specific areas.

C. Ask parents to have the room safe for the next session. Remind parents that you will be conducting another HAPI-R observation at the following session.

D. *Remind the parent that although the home is much safer for her or his children, there is no substitute for parental supervision.* The safest of homes can pose any number of risks to children left unsupervised.

E. Give positive feedback to parents for identifying and removing hazards and taking steps to ensure that their home is as safe as possible for their family.

Sessions 2–4

These sessions involve continuing to identify and remove hazards in the remaining rooms of the home. The format of each session is essentially the same, so they have been condensed here to save space. Be sure that all hazards are removed in previously trained rooms before moving on to training in other rooms. For example, before beginning training in the second room, all hazards in the first room in which training was conducted should have been addressed. Before conducting training in the third room, all hazards in the first and second rooms should have been addressed. This may mean that the number of sessions increases to allow sessions in which training in previously targeted rooms continues without addressing any of the hazards in a new room. This will depend on the number and degree of hazards, on the amenability of the family to removing these hazards, and on the initiative the family takes in removing hazards.

I. Conduct a HAPI-R and CLEAN observation for each room before beginning training.

II. Review the material covered at the previous session.

A. Dimensions of cleanliness

1. Clean/dirty

2. Clothes and linens not belonging

3. Other objects not belonging

B. Three ways to make hazards inaccessible

1. Use child-resistant closures

2. Lock up items

3. Place items out of child's reach

C. The eight categories of hazards (see definitions in section on HAPI-R assessment)

> > D. How to determine if hazards are accessible
> > E. Ask parent to restate as much of the information as possible.
> > F. Prompt information parent forgets.
> > G. Check for questions.
> III. Review parent's hazard removal and cleaning since previous session and provide positive feedback for corrections made.
> > A. Ask parent to tell you about the hazards and areas in need of cleaning that remained after the previous session and give them an opportunity to tell and show what they did to remove the hazards (previous week's assignments). This review should be conducted for all rooms in which training has previously been conducted, not just the room targeted during the previous session. This is to ensure that parents not only remove the hazards but also keep their home safe after several weeks.
> > B. Provide specific positive feedback to parents for removing hazards from and cleaning item areas in the rooms in which training has already taken place and for maintaining a clean, safe home.
> > > 1. If all hazards have been made inaccessible and all item areas are clean, praise parent and encourage her or him to maintain at that level.
> > > 2. If hazards remain:
> > > > a. Praise parent for any improvements over previous week's score.
> > > > b. Help the parent to locate areas in which hazards remain and item areas in need of cleaning.
> > > > c. Have parent correct a few items. Provide positive feedback.
> > > > d. Provide instructions and suggestions about making any remaining hazards inaccessible. If possible, ask parent to address these remaining hazards at this time. Only if it is not possible to address these hazards at this time (because special tools or safety accessories are needed), ask the parent to address these hazards during the following week before your next visit to the home. Remind them that the longer hazards remain, the greater the likelihood that their children may be harmed.
> > > > e. If parents need additional assistance in removing hazards, offer your help. This may involve locating additional safety devices or tools, providing assistance installing safety devices, or helping them contact apartment managers or property owners to make repairs.
> IV. Begin locating areas in need of cleaning and removing hazards.
> > A. Determine the room in which training will be conducted (based on which room poses the greatest hazards) and discuss with the parent whether it is a good day for working in that particular room.
> > B. Give specific feedback about CLEAN score in this room.
> > > 1. Identify one item area. Parents should be able to identify areas in need of cleaning after several sessions. Gradually shift this responsibility from yourself to the parent in such a way that the parent can successfully identify cleanliness problems and describe how they can best be cleaned.
> > > 2. Review definitions for dimensions of cleanliness and provide specific feedback and instructions for that area.

C. Help parent clean the item area.
   1. Discuss methods to improve cleanliness of the area.
   2. Model methods if necessary.
   3. Identify other item areas and provide specific feedback. Again, parents should be able to identify these areas as training progresses.
   4. Give parent assignment to complete remaining item areas before next session.
D. Provide feedback.
   1. Verbal, descriptive praise (for example, "Great, you organized all of the papers that were on this table.")
   2. Suggestions (e.g., "In order to clean that area, you might neatly fold and stack the clothes.")
E. Give specific feedback about HAPI score for that room (that is, "I have found hazards in 3 of the categories of hazards, and we will begin to remove each of these hazards today").
   1. Describe the eight categories of hazards and how these hazards could endanger the lives of small children (refer to the HAPI-R assessment definitions given earlier in this chapter). This discussion should be focused on specific hazards within the current room rather than focusing discussion on every category of hazard in a generic fashion.
   2. Identify specific subcategories of hazards that are present in the current room.
   3. Review the three methods to make hazards inaccessible.
F. Help the parent locate one hazard and demonstrate how it could be made inaccessible by one of the three methods. As training progresses, parents should be able to do this with less and less prompting. You should gradually decrease your prompting in such a way that the parent succeeds in identifying hazards and describing how they can be decreased.
   1. Describe the hazard and different strategies for making it inaccessible.
   2. When necessary, demonstrate how to use childproof devices such as drawer latches or cabinet locks.
G. Have parent practice identifying and removing remaining hazards.
   1. Ask parent to locate a similar item.
   2. Ask parent to make hazard inaccessible.
   3. Provide feedback:
      a. Verbal, descriptive praise (for example, "Good, you have placed the matches way up high and out of your child's reach").
      b. Suggestions (for example, "In order to make that item inaccessible, you will need to put it in a place where there is no furniture a child can climb on to reach it").
H. Continue to locate *all* hazardous items throughout the room.
   1. Model strategies for making items inaccessible.
   2. Ask the parent to practice these strategies until all hazards have been identified and addressed.
   3. Continue to provide feedback.
V. *End the session.*
A. At the end of the session, review any hazards that remain.

B. Ask the parent to correct all hazards. If necessary, leave a checklist of specific hazards or areas to remind parents of the hazard and how it can be made inaccessible. With some families, it may be necessary to devise more creative strategies to prompt them to remove hazards and to continue to ensure that each room is safe. These strategies might include individualized checklists or charts or the use of Polaroid photographs to highlight specific areas. Over time, as appropriate, less prompting should be used. Parents should be encouraged and praised for locating and removing hazards independently.

C. *Remind the parent that although the home is much safer for her or his children, there is no substitute for parental supervision.* The safest of homes can pose any number of risks to children left unsupervised.

D. Ask parents to have the room in which training was just conducted safe for the next session. Remind parents that you will be conducting another HAPI-R and CLEAN observation at the following session.

E. Give positive feedback to parents for identifying and removing hazards and taking steps to ensure that their home is as safe as possible for their family.

Session 5

This session is labeled Session 5, but depending on the number of sessions a particular family needs, training may be completed earlier or may take several more sessions than have been outlined here. The best determinations of the point at which training is complete are the HAPI-R and CLEAN scores for each room. The training criterion is always zero hazards, but it may be appropriate for a home in which there are no infants or toddlers to retain a very small number of hazards. For example, a family in which there are no children under age 5 or 6 may choose to leave bottles of shampoo and conditioner on a lower shelf in the shower, as it is unlikely that most children over this age would ingest these substances. This is an individual decision and should be discussed among you and the family in each case to ensure that homes are appropriately safe for the children living in that home.

Session 5, the final session, is not necessarily a training session. Instead, the training is briefly reviewed, and any other remaining hazards that need to be addressed are identified. Counselors and parents may engage in discussion of how parents can maintain a safe and clean home. Although initially removing hazards from the home might pose many challenges for some families, it is more likely that maintaining a safe home after training is complete is a larger challenge.

This session may also involve looking to the future and anticipating possible hazards that may become a problem in the future. For instance, as children grow, their reach and eye level also grow. This means that areas that may have been inaccessible in one year will become accessible in the coming years. Kitchen and bathroom counters may have been out of reach, but as the children grow, they may be able to reach knives left on the counter or vitamins or cosmetics left near the bathroom sink. Cabinet doors and drawers a child was not able to open as a toddler may become easier to open as that child becomes bigger and stronger. This means that drawer and cabinet latches may be needed.

    I. Conduct a HAPI-R and CLEAN observation for each room.

   II. Review the material covered at the previous session.

      A. Dimensions of cleanliness

         1. Clean/dirty

         2. Clothes and linens not belonging

         3. Other objects not belonging

      B. Three ways to make hazards inaccessible

         1. Use child-resistant closures

         2. Lock up items

         3. Place items out of child's reach

      C. The eight categories of hazards (see definitions in section on HAPI-R assessment)

      D. How to determine if hazards are accessible

      E. Ask parent to restate as much of the information as possible.

      F. Prompt information parent forgets.

      G. Check for questions.

  III. Review the previous training sessions and highlight the important changes the parent has made in the home. Offer praise and congratulations that she or he has made the home safe and clean for the children.

  IV. Remind the parent that although the home is much safer for the children, there is no substitute for parental supervision. The safest of homes can pose any number of risks to children left unsupervised.

   V. Problem solve strategies for maintaining a clean and safe home, such as setting aside time each week to clean, checking for hazards periodically, checking to assure that childproof latches and locks are used appropriately, and always supervising children regardless of where they are in the home and what they are doing.

  VI. Anticipate how the home conditions will need to change over time to accommodate the children's growth and development. Although items that may pose a risk to an infant may not be hazardous for a 5-year-old, as that child grows, his or her height will make some areas that were previously inaccessible now accessible.

 VII. Give positive feedback to parents for identifying and removing hazards and taking steps to ensure that their home is as safe as possible for their family. Congratulate the parent on the hard work just completed, and thank the parents for allowing you to look throughout their home.

VIII. Give parent a Consumer Satisfaction Questionnaire.

      A. In order to determine how acceptable the assessment and training procedures were for parents, they should be asked to fill out a Consumer Satisfaction Questionnaire. (See Appendix 4.12 for the form used in Project SafeCare. This form may be adapted to suit the needs of other programs.)

      B. Request that parents fill out survey items as honestly as possible, as the program will benefit from their opinions and feedback.

      C. Parents should be asked to complete the survey independently and return it to you at the next appointment or by mail.

COMMON PROBLEMS AND SOLUTIONS

One frequent problem that is encountered in safety and cleanliness training is that, although it is necessary to actually look through homes to identify examples of hazards within homes, it can seem intrusive, awkward, and uncomfortable to families. In Project SafeCare, every effort was made to convey our understanding of this to families and to ensure that parents were comfortable with how much counselors actually saw. Before conducting any observations, and after fully explaining what assessment and training involved, the counselor and parent read and discussed the Home Safety and Cleanliness Participant Consent form. Parents had the option to make any area off-limits at this time, as well as at any time throughout assessment and training. Parents were always made aware in advance of sessions in which home safety and cleanliness would be addressed. Before beginning each assessment, the counselors asked permission to look through the home, and parents were invited to be present during the observation. In many cases, parents became comfortable with the assessment and went about other business while the counselors completed the observation. As discussed earlier in this chapter, counselors were always very aware of the impact of their presence and actions on the family. They were always aware of how it might feel to have others looking through their own homes for hazardous or cluttered conditions. In some cases, however, some parents did not want to participate in this component. Parents always had the option to withdraw from this training component. In this case, the counselor acknowledged the parents' request, asked if she or he might still discuss home safety and cleanliness, and provided some tips for making the home safe for young children. In this case, the extensive assessment was not conducted as described, but rather the training was conducted in such a way that only the most easily observed hazards were addressed, such as those on the kitchen counter or the coffee table. Parents were still provided with safety latches to install on cabinets and drawers. The counselor emphasized that the reason for conducting the assessments and training was to ensure that the home was safe for their young children. Looking at the home from the children's eye level for every type of hazard present can reduce the risk for accidents or injuries.

Another common problem was maintenance of the changes families made in their homes. In families experiencing multiple stressors, home cleanliness and safety may not be of a high priority on a daily basis. The goal of training is to change the home environment in such a way that keeping the home safe and clean is made simpler. In some cases, however, these changes are difficult to maintain. Many families demonstrated exemplary maintenance of significant reductions in hazards, but for some families, this was difficult. During training, the importance of continually monitoring the home for hazards is emphasized. As children grow, they become more mobile and have greater access to a wide variety of hazardous conditions. The counselor and parent discussed strategies to anticipate this and to make their home safe for their growing children.

Families living in poor conditions, such as in overcrowded homes or in poorly maintained homes or apartments, may not have the financial resources to purchase safety latches or locked containers for securing hazards. In these cases, it would be helpful to provide some of these materials to the family or to gain the support of local businesses or other agencies that can donate these items or money to purchase them. In some cases, it may be necessary to assist the family in contacting rental agencies or landlords to obtain needed repairs to the home. If windows do not have screens or the walls have paint that is peeling, offer assistance to the family in seeing that these repairs are completed by the property owners or maintenance staff. This process will be helpful in modeling advocacy and assertiveness skills to families.

Finally, families were frequently observed to be living with other relatives, friends, or roommates. This poses a challenge because families do not have sole control over their living environment and may have to ask others living in the home to cooperate in making the home safe. It may be suggested to families that others living in the home be invited to participate in training if the parents agree to do so. If a good relationship exists between the family and others in the home, this may not pose a problem in conducting training. In some cases, however, the relationship between the family and others in the home may not be a good one. It then becomes important to discuss this situation in private with the family and to come up with some way to reduce accessible hazards and to improve the cleanliness of the home while working with others in the home.

CASE EXAMPLE

Jerry was a 39-year-old father of a 2-year-old daughter, Janine. He was reported for child neglect by neighbors who could see that the child was often unattended and that the home was extremely dirty and in disarray. The family lived with Jerry's mother, Sylvia, who had many pets, such as cats, birds, and rabbits. Although the animal cages were kept in the living room, the animals were allowed to roam freely through the house. Animal droppings, food, and hair could be found on all surfaces throughout the living room, dining room, and kitchen. In addition, because Jerry and Janine had recently moved into Sylvia's small home, the house was cluttered with personal belongings, papers, boxes, and other assorted items. The house was very dirty, cluttered, and extremely crowded. Even if Jerry and his mother had attempted to clean the home, there was very little space in which to store their belongings. After several sessions with Jerry in which health training was conducted, the counselors continued to develop rapport with Jerry and his mother, even though Sylvia was not actively participating in training. It was extremely important to include Sylvia to the extent that she wanted to be included, because it would later be necessary to work with her to make her home clean and safe for her granddaughter. During the first few sessions, Jerry had reported to the counselors that moving back in with his mother had placed a strain on their relationship and that he was reluctant to make any changes to her home without her permission.

After several sessions, the counselors brought up the topic of home safety and cleanliness with both Jerry and Sylvia in such a way as not to be offensive. The emphasis was placed on Janine's increasing ability to move freely about the house and the need to make her surroundings safe. The counselors explained the rationale for conducting home safety and cleanliness observations and how they would be conducted. They emphasized that the family could move about the home with the counselors as they conducted the observations and could specify any areas that were off-limits.

After several home safety and cleanliness observations during which counselors assessed the kitchen, dining room, living room, bathroom, and the child's bedroom, it was determined that training would begin in the living room, which was the most cluttered room and the room in which Janine spent most of her time. Home safety and cleanliness training were conducted concurrently, with item areas, or small, discrete areas within each room, being used to divide rooms into smaller, more manageable areas. Because the room was so cluttered and the family had such limited storage space, it was important to break down the job of cleaning and making the home safe into smaller, more manageable tasks.

Initially, the counselor described how to determine which areas were accessible to Janine based on her height and reach. They also discussed the categories of hazards and the dimensions of cleanliness. Then the counselor and the family began with only one item area, the couch and side tables in the living room. They identified hazards and how they could be eliminated using one of the three methods (latches, locks, and placing items out of the child's reach). For example, bottles of pet medications were placed on the top shelf of a cupboard with a childproof latch. Matches and lighters were placed on a shelf that was out of Janine's reach. The counselor showed the father and grandmother how to determine that the height of this shelf was out of the child's reach and to ensure that she could not climb onto adjacent furniture and then obtain these hazardous items. They also identified how the item area could be cleaned, such as by picking up stacks of mail and papers that were cluttering the tables, putting away clothes that had been on the couch for several weeks, and wiping down the tables with a cleaner. When necessary, the counselor modeled how these steps should be conducted. The counselor completed these steps initially, but as training progressed, the counselor gradually prompted the family to identify problem areas and strategies for removing hazards. Eventually, Jerry and Sylvia were doing most of the work, and the counselor was just prompting and providing feedback.

Many of the changes that were to be made were time-consuming or required purchasing storage supplies, such as a locking cabinet or boxes that could be locked or childproof latched. Jerry and Sylvia were asked to purchase a locking cabinet in which to store food and supplies for the animals. Childproof latches were provided for the family to install on all kitchen and bathroom cupboards and drawers containing hazards. They were asked to place all hazardous items they had previously left out in the open into these latched cabinets. Jerry and Sylvia were able to make many of these changes themselves without the physical assistance of the counselors, so after each item area was discussed, the strategies Jerry and Sylvia were going to use were written down. After Jerry and Sylvia went through each item area, removed some of the hazards while the counselors were present, and made a list of what still needed to be done, the counselor asked Jerry and Sylvia to complete these tasks before the following session. Each session was conducted similarly, with less time spent discussing safety and cleanliness strategies after the initial session. Each remaining session was dedicated to one specific room, but before beginning training, the counselor conducted safety and cleanliness observations in every room to determine if conditions were improving. If hazards remained, additional feedback was provided to ensure that the hazards would be removed prior to the next session. At the final session, the counselor went through the entire home with Jerry and Sylvia, praising their efforts, providing additional prompts when necessary, and planning how the home could be kept safe and clean in the future. Specific attention was given to strategies that would need to be implemented as Janine grew up. Her height and reach would change, so that she would soon be able to reach areas that had previously been inaccessible. Throughout training, the counselor emphasized that, although the home was becoming safer, there is never any substitute for parental supervision. The importance of always supervising Janine's activities was explained to Jerry and Sylvia.

Following each training session, Jerry and Sylvia's home became increasingly safe and clean. They rearranged their home so that the items that made their home hazardous and cluttered were organized and placed in child-safe containers. They moved some of the animals to provide a safer play area for Janine, and, over time, they continued to maintain a clean home. Although the number of total hazards throughout their home had been well over 100 in each room, training resulted in dramatic decreases in these hazards. After several training sessions, they even had begun to remove hazards in rooms that had not yet been targeted for training. By the time training was complete, there were no accessible hazards in any of the rooms of their home. Their home had a clean and neat appearance and provided a safe and enjoyable environment for the family. Several months after this training program was complete, these improvements were maintained. There was never any indication that this training program caused more friction between Jerry and his mother. In fact, they appeared to be getting along very well after working together to make their home safe for Janine.

Home Safety and Cleanliness Assessment Participant Consent

One of the areas we will be focusing on is home safety and maintenance. By providing a clean and safe home, your children will grow up in an environment that is healthy and will help their development. A cleanliness checklist (CLEAN) and a Home Accident Prevention Inventory (HAPI-R) have been designed to help point out any problem areas or safety hazards that may exist in your home. A counselor will look around areas of your home using these checklists. You may accompany the counselor throughout your home at any time during this activity. The counselor may also want to measure your child's height to help determine if certain areas of the home are out of your child's reach.

If you do not wish a Project SafeCare counselor to look in certain areas of your home, please place an "X" in the blank next to that area listed below.

Living Room _____
Look in furniture cabinets? _____
Look in furniture drawers? _____
Look under furniture? _____
Look behind furniture? _____
Other? Please list below: _____

_____

Bathroom _____
Look in medicine cabinets? _____
Look in cabinets? _____
Look in drawers? _____
Other? Please list below: _____

_____

Kitchen _____
Look in cabinets? _____
Look in drawers? _____
Look in refrigerator
    and freezer? _____
Other? Please list below: _____

_____

Bedrooms _____
Look in cabinets? _____
Look in drawers? _____
Look under bed? _____
Look in closets? _____
Other? Please list below: _____

_____

Miscellaneous _____
Look in boxes? _____
Look at personal or household products? _____
Other? Please list below: _____

_____

I have read, or had read to me, the above. I agree to and understand the home cleanliness and safety procedure. I further understand that I can revoke this consent at anytime.

_____   _____
Parent   Date

_____   _____
Counselor   Date

Home Accident Prevention Inventory— Revised Data Sheet

Family _____   Date _____

Child _____   Session # _____

Observer _____   Eye level _____   Reach _____

Bl = Baseline
T = Training
F = Follow-up
A/A + D = agreements divided by agreements + disagreements

Room							
Condition (Bl T F)							
	Number of Hazards		Total	A/A + D	Number of Hazards	Total	A/A + D
Poison by Solids & Liquids							
Pill meds (w/o safety caps)							
Tube meds							
Inhaler meds							
Liquid meds							
Deodorizers							
Jar meds							
Detergents & cleansers							
Polishes & waxes							
Alcoholic beverages							
Beauty products							
Insecticides & rodenticides							
Paints & stains							
Solvents & thinners							
Glues & adhesives							
Petroleum products							
Fertilizers & herbicides							
Poisonous plants							
Fire & Electrical Hazards							
Combustibles							
Protective appliance covers							
Fireplaces w/o screens							
Outlet/switch w/o plates							
Electrical cords/plugs							

(continued)

	Number of Hazards			Total	A/A + D	Number of Hazards			Total	A/A + D
Suffocation by Mech. Objects										
Plastics										
Crib cords										
Small Objects										
Ingestible small objects										
Sharp Objects										
Sharp objects										
Firearms										
Firearms										
Falling Hazards										
Balconies										
Steps										
Windows										
Drowning Hazards										
Bathtubs/sinks										
Buckets										
Wading pools										
				/					/	
					%					%

Open garbage? _____

Spoiled food? _____

Checklist for Living Environments to Assess Neglect Data Sheet

Family _____ Room _____ Observer _____ Session # _____ Phase: Bl T F Date _____

+ – 0

Item Area	Points	10	0
	Rating	Clean	Dirty

Clean/Dirty

Total points

Number of Clothes and Linens

5	4	3	2	1	0
0	1–5	6–10	11–15	16–20	20+

Number of Objects Not Belonging

5	4	3	2	1	0	Total Points
0	1–5	6–10	11–15	16–20	20+	

NOTE: Can use side or bottom total column, but not both.

Comments:

Agreement scores:
Divide number of agreements by agreements
plus disagreements, and then multiply by 100.
Agree = _____
Agree + Disagaree = _____
(A/A+D) x 100 = _____

Total Ratings = _____
No. of item areas = _____
Divide total ratings by no.
of item areas = _____ / 20 = _____ × 100 = _____

Home Safety and Cleanliness Consumer Satisfaction Questionnaire

Thank you for participating in the home safety and cleanliness services provided by Project SafeCare. We would like to learn some of your thoughts and feelings about the program. Please read the following comments and circle the answer that best describes your feelings about each statement. Please be as honest as possible. Your responses will be kept confidential and will be useful to project staff in improving the services we provide. Thank you for your time and cooperation.

1. Since I have completed the safety and cleanliness program, my home is:

Much safer	Safe	No different	Less safe	Much less safe
1	2	3	4	5

2. Conducting the safety program in other homes where small children live would be a:

Very good idea	Good idea	Neither good nor bad idea	Bad idea	Very bad idea
1	2	3	4	5

3. I am better able to identify safety hazards in my home.

Strongly agree	Agree	Neutral	Disagree	Strongly disagree
1	2	3	4	5

4. I am better able to clean my home and keep it clean.

Strongly agree	Agree	Neutral	Disagree	Strongly disagree
1	2	3	4	5

5. While having the individual who conducted the training look through my home, I felt:

Very comfortable	Somewhat comfortable	Neither comfortable nor uncomfortable	Somewhat uncomfortable	Very uncomfortable
1	2	3	4	5

6. How much time did it take to make your home safe and clean for the children?

Almost no time	Very little	Some	A lot	Too much time
1	2	3	4	5

7. From now on I plan to follow the recommendations of the safety and cleanliness program:

Always	Most of the time	Sometimes	Seldom	Never
1	2	3	4	5

(continued)

8. The safety devices I was given, such as locks for my cabinets, were:

Very useful	Useful	Neither useful nor useless	Useless	Very useless
1	2	3	4	5

9. The amount of effort required to make my home safe and clean for children was acceptable.

Strongly agree	Agree	Neutral	Disagree	Strongly disagree
1	2	3	4	5

10. I feel that the safety program provided me with new and useful skills for making hazards inaccessible.

Strongly agree	Agree	Neutral	Disagree	Strongly disagree
1	2	3	4	5

11. I believe that the home safety program failed to address all of the hazards accessible to my children in my home.

Strongly agree	Agree	Neutral	Disagree	Strongly disagree
1	2	3	4	5

12. Since the training program, my child has been involved in a household accident (i.e., swallowing a poisonous substance, being burned or shocked):

Never	Once	Twice	Three times	Four or more times
1	2	3	4	5

Rate how useful each of these items was in helping you benefit from the services you received, if relevant.

	Useful	Somewhat useful	OK	Slightly useful	Useless
1. Counselor's explanations					
2. Counselor's demonstrations					
3. Practice during sessions					
4. Practice outside of sessions					
5. Counselor's feedback					
6. Safety supplies					

(continued)

131

Please rate the counselor who conducted the safety and cleanliness training program.

	Strongly agree	Agree	Neutral	Disagree	Strongly disagree
1. Was warm and friendly					
2. Was helpful					
3. Gave clear explanations					
4. Was knowledgeable					
5. Was negative or critical					
6. Treated me fairly					
7. Was willing to spend extra time when I needed it					
8. Kept our scheduled appointments					
9. Was on time to scheduled appointments					
10. Spent too much time looking around my home					

Comments:

7

Infant and Child Health Care Skills

Families reported for or at risk for child maltreatment may lack the skills needed to provide adequate health and medical care to their infants and children. This lack of care may increase the likelihood that medical conditions will remain undetected or untreated or that health conditions may contribute to continued maltreatment (NRC, 1993). For example, a cold, flu, or ear infection may lead to bacterial infections, pneumonia, or even hearing loss. Complications from a runny nose may lead to a secondary sinus infection (Fries & Vickery, 1990). Children who are neglected are thus at risk for serious health problems that can adversely affect future health and development (NRC, 1993).

Infant and child health care training was offered to provide parents with the skills necessary to identify symptoms and provide appropriate treatment. Although it was provided to parents who were at risk and reported for child maltreatment, the skills described here are applicable for all parents and care providers. These procedures were adapted from those described by Delgado and Lutzker (1988) and have been evaluated and refined in Project SafeCare with families at risk for and reported for child maltreatment (Bigelow & Lutzker, 2000)

In the five-session training protocol described here, parents are taught to identify and record their child's symptoms, to refer to a health manual to determine a course of treatment, and then to either consult a physician, seek emergency treatment, or treat the symptoms at home. Parents are also taught to continue to monitor symptoms and to provide additional treatment as needed. Although this protocol requires parents to read and write, a number of parents have been taught to follow a set of general steps and then to consult friends or family members to assist in determining the course of treatment by consulting the health manual. Additional skills taught throughout the course of the training sessions include taking a temperature, administering medications, and taking a pulse.

The following sections outline the materials used during child health care training, the assessment and training protocol, and case examples to illustrate their application.

HEALTH CARE TRAINING MATERIALS

Parents were provided with materials that they were to keep for future use. All materials were available in English and Spanish. Most of these materials can be found in the appendices, although due to space limitations, some materials have been excluded, such as the health manual provided to parents and the full set of health care scenarios. A complete set of materials and a set of the Spanish-language materials may be obtained by contacting the authors. Parents were provided with a health manual and symptom guide, Parent Behavior Checklist, Health Recording Chart, and health supplies for use at each training and follow-up sessions. Parents were encouraged to refer to their materials when their children were ill and to keep their materials in a safe place so that they were available even after training was completed.

True/False Quizzes

Ten-item true–false quizzes are used to assess parents' knowledge of general health information. Six versions are available. The quizzes are administered at each assessment and training session unless parents complete 8 out of 10 items correctly on the first quiz. In this case, quizzes are administered only at the beginning and end of training and at subsequent follow-up assessment sessions. See Appendix 7.1 for an example of a true–false quiz.

Role-Play Scenario Cards

Scenario cards provide descriptions of scenarios in which children display a variety of symptoms characteristic of a particular illness or condition. Parents are presented these cards during a role-play scenario, in which their health care skills are observed. There are 19 scenarios covering a range of illnesses and conditions. Scenarios are depicted on index cards that are either presented to the parent or from which the counselor reads to the parent. For example, one such scenario states, "Your 1-year-old child has been cranky and whiny all afternoon. His/her nose has been running, and you notice he/she has been sneezing all day long. During the night, your child wakes up coughing. When you check, you notice that he/she is very warm."

On being presented with a role-play scenario card, parents are asked to tell the counselor what they believe the problem is and to show the counselor exactly how they would go about treating the symptoms. There are four categories of role-play scenarios, designated by the type of treatment called for. The four types of treatments are: treat at home, call the doctor, seek emergency treatment, and a combination of treating at home, then calling the doctor. See Appendix 7.2 for a list of illnesses covered in the role-play scenarios and Appendix 7.3 for sample scenario cards.

Scenario Answer Sheets

Role-play scenario answer sheets contain a list of responses that counselors are to provide to parents throughout each role-play scenario, such as what a child's temperature is and what symptoms are after the initial treatment. Answers are provided for correct and incorrect responses. Parents do not see these answer sheets. See Appendix 7.4 for sample scenario answer sheets.

Health Manual

The health manual was adapted from home medical handbooks (Fries & Vickery, 1990; Stoppard, 1986) and consists of five sections: "Using References," "Planning and Prevention," "Caring for Your Child at Home," "Calling the Doctor," and "Urgent Care." Due to space limitations, these materials could not be included here. Published health manuals available in bookstores may be adapted for your own use. It is important that the manual provide information similar to what is described here, especially step by step instructions for treating a variety of child health issues.

Symptom and Illness Guide

The symptom and illness guide is presented to parents as part of the health manual. It describes symptoms and treatments for 35 illnesses or conditions. For each, the following information is provided: whether a condition is serious, whether the illness should be treated at home or by a physician, instructions for what a parent should do to treat the illness, and what a physician might do to treat the illness. See Appendix 7.5 for a list of the symptoms and illnesses discussed in this manual.

Parent Behavior Checklist

The Parent Behavior Checklist consists of the steps involved in identifying illnesses, treating at home, calling the physician, and seeking emergency treatment. This list consists of 25 items that function as the primary task analysis and measure of parents' health care skills. Counselors record completed steps during the role-play scenarios on the counselor's version of this task analysis. The counselor's version of this checklist includes a set of boxes across from each step in which counselors check off correct steps. The parent's version is slightly different in that the steps are stated from the parent's point of view and that there is only one set of boxes in which to check off completed steps. See Appendix 7.6 for the counselor's version and Appendix 7.7 for the parent's version. Then see Appendix 7.8 for operational definitions for each step and scoring instructions for the Parent Behavior Checklist.

For each type of scenario—treat at home, call the doctor, emergency treatment, and treat at home first and then call the doctor—only applicable steps are scored during a role-play scenario. Thus, for example, in an emergency scenario, parents are required to state the problem and seek emergency treatment. When presented with a scenario requiring treatment at home, parents are required to complete all of the general steps (Section A on the counselor's checklist), and the treat-at-home steps (Section D). Scenarios involving calling the doctor involve the general steps (Section A) and the steps for calling the doctor (Section B). For scenarios calling for emergency treatment, parents are required only to state the problem (Section A, Item 1) and then seek emergency treatment (Section C). Steps that are not applicable to the role play being conducted are scored as "N/A" and are not included in the calculations of percentage correct.

Health Recording Chart

The Health Recording Chart is a worksheet on which parents record symptoms and treatments for one scenario or one occurrence of a child's illness. Space is provided in which parents can record symptoms and treatments and changes in symptoms over time. See Appendix 7.9 for a copy of the Health Recording Chart.

Health Supplies

Parents should have or be provided with a mercury thermometer, a medicine dropper, a medicine spoon, antibiotic ointment, bandages, gauze, first-aid tape, diaper cream, petroleum jelly, and cotton balls. A doll may be used during some sessions in order to simulate administering medication or taking a temperature when it is inappropriate to do so with the child or when the child is not present.

The content of the symptom and illness guide, the Health Recording Chart, and the list of recommended medical supplies included in the health manual was validated by 11 physicians and family practice medical residents. Comments provided by these health care professionals were incorporated into the development of these materials.

ASSESSMENT SESSIONS

Parents' child health care skills are assessed in two ways. Parent behavior is assessed through observation of their behavior in a role-play situation using the Parent Behavior Checklist, whereas parent knowledge, which does not always translate into actual skills, is assessed by the use of true–false quizzes. To assess parents' health care skills most accurately, you should directly observe those skills when parents are treating children's illnesses. Parents' health care skills, however, are most frequently demonstrated at times when observation is not possible, so asking parents to demonstrate these skills in a role-play situation provides this opportunity. Assessment takes place over several sessions, and generally three role-play scenarios are conducted prior to beginning training.

Role-Play Scenarios

Prior to health care skills training, parents are asked to respond as they normally would in a role-play situation to a scenario in which a child is described as demonstrating symptoms of an illness or injury. After instructions on how the role-play scenarios are to be conducted, parents are presented with a role-play scenario card. The scenario card is either shown to the parent or read aloud, depending on parents' preference. The parent is then instructed to pretend that the child described in the scenario is his or her child, tell the observer what he or she thinks the illness is, and show the observer everything that he or she would do to treat the symptoms. The counselor provides additional prompts to the parent as they proceed through the role-play scenario. In order to provide a broad indication of the parent's skill level, a number of scenarios are conducted over several sessions. In most cases, at least three scenarios are administered.

Counselors do not provide feedback to the parent other than the prompts provided on the role-play scenario answer sheet corresponding to the scenario given to the parent. During training, feedback is provided after the scenario is completed, but no feedback is provided during the baseline, or pretraining, phase. The counselor explains that the purpose of the role-play scenarios is to find out what parents would normally do when presented with these situations. They should do whatever they believe is the best thing to do in the situation. This provides a baseline against which to compare the effects of the health skill training program. The scenarios involve checking symptoms several hours later, and, in these cases, the counselor provides minimal prompts necessary to determine when parents check symptoms and how they respond if the symptoms improve, get worse, or stay the same. To illustrate using the scenario previously described (the 1-year-old child), if the parent initially indicated that he or she would give the child the appropriate dosage of children's acetaminophen in response to a fever of 100.8 degrees and then check the child's temperature later, the counselor would state that the child's temperature had decreased to 98 degrees. The parent would be asked again to demonstrate what she or he would do in this situation.

If at any point the parent demonstrates incorrect treatment of the illness, the counselor provides responses that continue the role play. For example, if a parent indicates that she or he would call the physician when the correct response was to treat at home, the observer plays the role of the physician during a phone call and instructs the parent in the correct at-home treatment. The counselor as the physician in the role play provides only specific instructions in how to treat the symptoms at home. The parent is not told that she should have avoided calling the physician. When parents indicate that they would call the physician when treating at home was the preferred response, the corresponding item on the task analysis is scored as incorrect.

The percentage correct on successive role-play scenarios is graphed on a weekly basis in order to track the parent's progress throughout the training sessions. Generally, there is a gradual increase in percentage correct throughout the five training sessions, and the majority of parents meet the 100% mastery criterion by the fifth training session, if not earlier. In Project SafeCare, it was rare that parents would not meet this criterion for each type of role-play scenario because of the very precise and simple way in which the target skills were presented to parents in this package.

Steps for Conducting a Role-Play Scenario

1. Choose the role-play scenario to administer. During assessment, the parent should be presented with each type of scenario.
2. Give the parent the following instructions:

"Read [or listen] carefully. When you [I]have read the scenario card, I want you to *show* me what you would do for the problem described. Start by telling me what you think the problem is, then do whatever you would normally do. You can show me with your child or with the doll."

3. Give the parent the scenario card or read the scenario card to the parent.
4. Tell the parent to *tell* you what she or he thinks the problem is and *show* you what she or he would do in that situation.
5. If the parent *tells* you what she or he would do, say that you really need to *see* her *doing* it and ask her or him to *show* you.
6. If the parent says she or he would take a temperature, tell her or him to *show* you how she or he would do that. If the parent says she or he would administer medication, tell her or him to *show* you the medication and how she or he would administer it but to not really administer it.
7. If the parent says she or he would call the doctor, emergency room, or a friend, tell him or her to *show* you and say that you will play the part of the person on the other end of the telephone. Refer to the scenario answer card for instructions for role playing telephone calls.
8. If the parent indicates that she or he would check on symptoms again in the future or readminister medicine or treatment at some future time, ask her or him to tell you when (specifically), then indicate that the time has elapsed and tell her or him to show you what she or he would do at that time. Refer to the scenario answer sheet for information to incorporate into role play for such situations.
9. If the parent chooses to treat the child at home, but does not specifically indicate that she or he would check symptoms again in the future, indicate that time has passed and tell the parent what symptoms are still present. Repeat until symptoms have been checked three times. If parent chooses to call the doctor or seek emergency treatment, score the behaviors already demonstrated and end the role play.
10. When the parent appears to be finished, ask if there is anything else she or he would do. If there is, tell her or him to show you. If there is nothing else that she or he would do, thank her or him for completing the role play.

Scoring the Role-Play Scenarios

1. For each step completed correctly, record a "+" in the appropriate space. For each step completed incorrectly or missed, record a "−" in the appropriate space. For steps that do not apply to the particular scenario, record "N/A" in the appropriate space. That is, if the scenario is "treat at home," score only the general steps and the treat-at-home steps. In this scenario, if a parent calls the doctor, score the treat-at-home steps "−" and the call-the-doctor and emergency-treatment steps "N/A."
2. Steps must be completed in the correct sequence in order to be scored correct (+).

That is, if the parent skips a step but later completes it correctly (but out of order), the step is scored as incorrect (–). If the parent skips a step but completes the next step correctly, the skipped step is scored incorrect (–). The completed step is scored correct (+). For example, if the parent administers cough syrup but failed to read the label until after she or he had administered the cough syrup, she or he would receive a "–" for the step labeled "Reads instructions on label for medication or in reference book." However, if she or he administered the cough syrup correctly (i.e., according to the instructions on the label), a "+" would be recorded for the step labeled "Follows instructions for administering treatment." The observer may need to read the label in order to determine whether the step was in fact performed correctly.

As an exception to this rule, if the parent must take the child's temperature in order to state the primary symptom (such as fever), the parent may complete Steps A2 and A3 (recording the symptoms on the chart and checking the manual) before correctly stating that the child has a fever. In this case, if the parent reports the correct symptoms, Step 1 ("states problem") would be scored as correct (+).

3. If the physician or the health manual recommends a treatment that requires supplies other than medicine or supplies not kept in a medicine cabinet, such as juice, liquids, bland foods, or ice, and the parent gets these supplies, score Step D1 ("gets recommended supplies from medicine cabinet") as correct (+).

4. If, while you are conducting a treat-at-home scenario, instructions on a label or in the manual indicate that a parent should talk to a doctor before administering the medicine the first time, *do not* score the steps for calling the doctor. Simply score Step D3 ("follows instructions for administering treatment") as you normally would. Role play the part of the physician and advise the parent to administer an appropriate dose.

5. When you are conducting a combined treat-at-home/call-the-doctor scenario, score Steps D1–D7, then score the steps for calling the doctor (Section B). Steps D8–D13 would be scored as "N/A." This is true even if the parent continues to treat the illness him- or herself.

6. If the information on the scenario answer sheet and in the health manual do not agree, use the information in the health manual to score the parent's behavior.

True/False Quizzes

Although not a primary measure of parent health care skills, true–false quizzes provide an indication of parents' knowledge of general health-related information. Six versions of the true–false quizzes are available, and each consists of 10 items. If a parent achieves 80% accuracy or greater on the initial true–false quiz during baseline, additional quizzes are not administered until the last session of health care skills training. This reduces the amount of time spent conducting assessments, an important consideration for parents who may be reluctant to participate in training. If a parent achieves less than 80% accuracy on the initial true–false quiz, additional quizzes are administered at subsequent sessions. True–false quizzes are also administered during follow-up observations.

Steps for Administering the True–False Quizzes:

1. Choose the quiz to be administered at the session. If the parent scores 80% or better on the first quiz, no more will be administered. If parent scores less than 80%, three more will be administered during assessment.
2. If the parent can read, give the quiz to the parent and ask her or him to read each statement and to indicate if the statement is true or false by circling "T" for true or "F" for false.
3. If the parent cannot read, read each statement to her or him and ask whether the statement is true or false. Record the response.

TRAINING PROCEDURES

Pretraining Assessment

In addition to the assessment of parents' skills before training, assessment continues during each training session in order to ensure that parents are, in fact, developing the target skills. The true–false quizzes are read to each parent aloud by the counselor, unless the parent indicates a preference to read the quiz silently. After the parent completes the quiz, a role-play scenario is conducted.

Written Materials

At the session before beginning training, the parent is provided with a binder containing the health manual and symptom guide and several copies of the Parent Behavior Checklist and the Health Recording Chart. The counselor briefly describes the format of the health manual and symptom guide, shows the Parent Behavior Checklist and Health Recording Chart to the parent but does not explain them, and asks the parent to read the first section of the health manual, "Using References," before the next session.

This phase of training is aimed at determining the effectiveness of providing written materials to parents without additional instruction or training. Assessment of the effectiveness of written materials alone consists of the one pretraining assessment scenario conducted on the first day of training prior to beginning health care skills instruction.

After conducting this training protocol with the large number of families who participated in Project SafeCare, it was apparent that the mere presentation of written materials failed to result in improvements in parent's health care skills. In other words, instructions, modeling, and repeated practice were required to achieve noticeable improvements in parent's health care skills. This is a very important point to remember.

Health Care Skills Training

Training is conducted in five sessions, with the first session including discussion and modeling of the steps of the Parent Behavior Checklist, followed by parent practice, and then a review of the "Using References" chapter of the health manual. Sessions 2, 3, and 4 involve additional practice on the steps of the Parent Behavior Checklist using novel role-play scenarios. During these sessions, parents are also taught basic child health care skills, such as how to take temperature and when and how parents should consult a physician and seek emergency treatment. Session 5 involves repeated practice using a number of role-play scenarios until parents meet the 100% correct mastery criterion. Table 7.1 provides a concise overview of the five sessions.

Immediately before each training session after the first one, a role-play scenario is administered to assess parent performance. Feedback on parent performance is provided after the role play is complete. The first training session involves a discussion of the steps of the task analysis and the rationale for health care skills training. Following this discussion, the counselor models the steps on the Parent Behavior Checklist using a role-play scenario. Parents are then prompted to practice the steps of the task analysis using the same role-play scenario. Following the parent's completion of this scenario, counselors provide feedback to the parent, praising the correct demonstration of the steps of the task analysis and providing corrective feedback for steps completed incorrectly. Feedback is provided only after the parent completes the scenario and includes a description of the steps the parents demonstrated correctly and prompts for how to improve performance. Counselors prompt the parents to practice again the steps completed incorrectly. Parents are not asked to practice steps previously completed correctly. During the first training session, the counselor and parent review the first section of the health manual, "Using References."

During Sessions 2 through 4, parents are provided with additional opportunities to practice the steps on the Parent Behavior Checklist in role-play scenarios. A novel role-play scenario is conducted to optimize parent's exposure to various child health care situations. Feedback is provided, and the counselor implements positive practice of the steps completed incorrectly following this role-play scenario. Sections 2 and 3 of the health manual, which discuss "Planning and Prevention" and "Caring for Your Child at Home," are reviewed during Training Sessions 2 and 3, respectively. During Session 4, Sections 4 and 5 of the manual, which discuss "Calling the Doctor" and "Urgent Care," are reviewed. For sections of the manual that contain instructions for specific skills, such as taking a temperature or administering medication, counselors describe and model these behaviors and then prompt parents to practice until each skill is completed correctly. These skills are practiced throughout the course of training as they appear in role-play scenarios. At the end of each session, parents are asked to read the following week's chapter or chapters. If the parent has not read the appropriate chapter before training sessions, the counselor reads over this material with the parent.

Throughout all five training sessions, parents are given the opportunity to ask questions about material presented in the manual and to practice the target skills. They are taught to keep records in their health manuals of such information as physician's telephone numbers, health insurance provider, or information sources. Further, they are also taught to take a temperature and pulse and to administer medications with a medicine dropper or spoon. At each session, parents are encouraged to use these newly learned skills in actual child care situations and to keep records of these incidents using the materials provided.

The fifth session consists of additional practice for each type of role-play scenario. The purpose of this session is to provide the parent with the opportunity to achieve the 100% mas-

TABLE 7.1. Infant and Child Health Care Skills Training Sessions

Session 1

    I. Pretraining assessment
   II. Describe rationale for Training Session 1
  III. Give parent health manual and extra Parent Behavior Checklists and Health Recording Charts
  IV. Review the Parent Behavior Checklist—Parent's Version
   V. Model steps of Parent Behavior Checklist
  VI. Ask parent to practice steps of Parent Behavior Checklist
 VII. Review the "Using References" section of health manual
VIII. End by reviewing, providing feedback, and asking parent to read "Planning and Prevention" section of the manual

Session 2

    I. Conduct a role-play scenario to assess parent performance
   II. Provide feedback to parent
  III. Make sure parent has health manual and extra Parent Behavior Checklists and Health Recording Charts
  IV. Describe rationale for Training Session 2
   V. Review material from previous session and answer any questions
  VI. Review Section 2 of health manual, "Planning and Prevention"
 VII. Provide feedback
VIII. Instructions, modeling, practice, and feedback
  IX. End the session by reviewing, providing feedback, and asking parent to read "Caring for Your Child at Home" section of the manual

Session 3

    I. Conduct a role-play scenario to assess parent performance
   II. Provide feedback to parent
  III. Make sure parent has health manual and extra Parent Behavior Checklists
  IV. Describe rationale for Training Session 3
   V. Review previous sessions and answer any questions
  VI. Review Section 3 of manual, "Caring for Your Child at Home"
 VII. Provide feedback
VIII. Instructions, modeling, practice, and feedback
  IX. End the session by reviewing, providing feedback, and asking parent to read "Calling the Doctor" and "Urgent Care" sections of the manual

Session 4

    I. Conduct a role-play scenario to assess parent performance
   II. Provide feedback to parent
  III. Make sure parent has health manual and extra Parent Behavior Checklists
  IV. Describe rationale for Training Session 4
   V. Review previous sessions questions
  VI. Review Sections 4 and 5 of the manual, "Calling the Doctor" and "Urgent Care"
 VII. Provide feedback
VIII. Instructions, modeling, practice, and feedback
  IX. End the session by reviewing, providing feedback, and explaining Session 5.

(continued)

TABLE 7.1. *(continued)*

<u>Session 5</u>

   I. Prepare materials in advance of session
  II. Describe rationale for Training Session 5
 III. Administer "treat at home" scenarios
 IV. Administer "call the doctor" scenarios
  V. Administer "emergency treatment" scenario
 VI. Determine if an additional session should be scheduled
VII. Review the session
VIII. End the session by giving feedback and encouraging the parent to keep the materials in a safe place and to continue to use them

tery criterion for each type of role play (treat at home, call the doctor, combined treat at home and then call the doctor, and emergency treatment). Practice continues until the parent performs 100% of all the steps correctly at least once for each of the three types of role plays, up to a maximum of three scenarios within each category of treatment (treat at home, call the doctor, and emergency treatment). Feedback and modeling are provided as needed after each role-play scenario when parents do not meet the mastery criterion. On occasions on which the parent does not perform 100% of the steps correctly on any one of the three opportunities, an additional session is scheduled to continue practice and feedback. The counselor emphasizes to parents who do not meet this criterion quickly that they should not feel worried or concerned. The scenarios provide a number of situations to which even the most experienced of parents would not know how to respond, and they should feel free to stop and ask questions at any time.

Steps for Conducting Health Care Skills Training

Session 1

The purpose of this session is to provide an introduction to and overview of training. Although the first session does not specifically address children's illnesses, it is a very important session in which the steps of the Parent Behavior Checklist and the information in the health manual and symptom guide are formally introduced.

   I. *Pretraining assessment.* Administer a novel role-play scenario before beginning training. The purpose of the pretraining observation is to assess the impact of written materials on the parent's behavior. Follow the protocol described in the "Assessment Sessions" section of this chapter when administering a role-play scenario. If the parent scores below 80% on any pretraining true–false quizzes, administer a novel quiz following the protocol previously described.

  II. *Rationale for training.* Describe the rationale for training. Include the following points:

- "You will learn ways to keep your child as healthy as possible."
- "You will learn to recognize when your child is ill."
- "You will learn how to care for your sick child at home."

- "You will learn how to know when it is time to call the doctor or seek emergency treatment."
- "You will learn how to use reference materials as a guide to caring for a sick child."
- "You will learn to follow steps that will be helpful for keeping good records of your child's health. Well-kept records of your child's health and health care will be useful each time you take him or her to the physician and when your child starts school."

III. Make sure parent has the health manual and extra Parent Behavior Checklists and Health Recording Charts.

IV. Review the Parent Behavior Checklist—Parent's Version.
   A. Tell the parent you will review the things a parent should do when her or his child is ill.
   B. Tell the parent that, although it may seem like there are a lot of steps, she or he will have many opportunities to practice and can always refer to the materials.
   C. Tell the parent that everything that you review in this session will be covered again in more detail in the rest of the training and is also covered in the manual.
   D. Explain the operational definitions and rationale for each step (see Appendix 7.8). Include the following points:"

   - "It is good to get in the habit of following a certain routine now while the child is well so that when he or she does get sick, you do not have to panic."
   - "Although some steps may seem repetitive or unnecessary, they will all prove to be important under certain circumstances. Thus, you should always try to follow all of them."
   - "The steps are designed so that following them is really the quickest way to figure out how to help your child feel better."
   - "The materials provide a place and a method for keeping good records of your child's health. You will need these when your child goes to school or child care."

   E. Answer any questions the parent may have.

V. Model the steps of the Parent Behavior Checklist.
   A. Tell the parent that you are going to demonstrate the steps.
   B. Ask her or him to score your performance using a copy of the Parent Behavior Checklist—Parent Version.
   C. Use a novel scenario and demonstrate the steps for a treat-at-home illness.

VI. Ask the parent to practice the steps of the Parent Behavior Checklist.
   A. Tell the parent that you would like her or him to practice the steps.
   B. Tell the parent that she or he may use any of the materials you have given her or him, including the manual and the checklist.
   C. Use the same scenario to improve the likelihood the parent will succeed. Instruct the parent to show you everything she or he would do.
   D. Score the parent's performance using the Parent Behavior Checklist—Counselor's Version.

E. Give feedback to parent. Provide descriptive praise for all steps performed correctly. By "descriptive praise" we mean praise of the behavior itself rather than just general praise. Thus say, "good job identifying that cough," rather than just saying, "good job." Identify the steps missed and instruct the parent about how to perform the steps correctly. Model the step or steps if necessary. Ask parent to repeat the missed steps and give feedback on practice.

VII. Review the "Using References" section of the health manual.

A. Identify the material for the parent by directing her or him to that section of the manual.

B. Ask the parent if she or he has read over this section before the session. (You will have asked her or him to do so at the end of the previous session.)

C. If she or he has read the section, answer any questions she or he has. Ask if she or he would like to read over any portion of this section together to make sure all of the material is understood. If so, read it again with the parent.

D. If the parent has not read the section, read the section aloud with her or him. Answer any questions.

E. Provide the parent with feedback regarding her or his reading of the assignment. Give descriptive praise or suggestions as needed. For example, "Great, you seemed to really understand that section," or "It might be helpful to write down any questions you think of while reading the materials."

VIII. End by reviewing the session, providing positive, descriptive feedback on the parent's performance, asking if there are any questions, and then asking the parent to read the section of the manual on "Planning and Prevention" before your next session.

Session 2

I. *Pretraining data collection.* If parent has not yet scored 80% or better on a true–false quiz, administer a new quiz. Administer a new treat-at-home scenario prior to beginning the training session.

II. Provide feedback to parent about performance.

A. Provide positive and descriptive praise.

B. Briefly review the steps missed.

C. Have parent practice the missed steps.

D. Give feedback on practice.

III. Make sure parent has the health manual and extra Parent Behavior Checklists and Health Recording Charts.

IV. Describe the rationale for Training Session 2.

- "You will learn to plan ahead for when your child is ill."
- "Planning ahead for preventing illness."

V. Briefly review the material covered in the previous session and answer any questions.

VI. Review Section 2 of the manual, "Planning and Prevention."

A. Direct the parent to the appropriate section in the manual.

B. Ask if she or he has had a chance to read it before the session.

C. If the parent has read the material, answer any questions the parent may have. Ask if she or he would like to read it again together to make sure the material is clearly understood. If so, then read it again with her or him.

D. If the parent has not read the material, read the section aloud with the parent and answer any questions.

VII. Provide the parent with feedback regarding her or his performance with the reading materials.

VIII. *Instructions, modeling, practice, and feedback.* Each skill should be discussed and modeled in its entirety for the parent. The parent should then be asked to practice the skill (either with a doll or with the child, when appropriate). Feedback should then be provided. Feedback should always begin by telling the parent the positive aspects of her or his performance. Then, if corrective feedback is necessary, simply explain the skills on which the parent needs more practice. Ask the parent to continue to practice steps not completed correctly, and provide assistance as necessary until the parent demonstrates the skills correctly.

A. Planning for sick days

1. Turn to the section of the health manual on "Planning for Sick Days" (a subsection of "Planning and Prevention").

2. Help the parent complete the forms in this section asking about names and phone numbers of people who can take care of her or his sick children if she or his is unable to stay home with them. Also included in this section are questions about child care center and school policies concerning children's illnesses, about financial or insurance information, and about emergency contact numbers.

3. Use problem-solving skills when necessary.

4. If parent does not have all the information necessary to complete the forms, ask her or him to find out the information before the next session.

5. Review the list of recommended health supplies for the home.

a. Identify supplies the parent already has.

b. Discuss with the parent how to get the remaining supplies.

c. Give any supplies that you provide to the parent.

B. Basics of good health

1. Turn to this section of the health manual (a subsection of "Planning and Prevention").

2. Review each of the items in the "Tips" box .

3. Discuss the parent's current practice regarding each item.

4. Discuss with the parent the items that she or he is currently not doing, if necessary.

C. About Nutrition

1. Turn to this subsection of the health manual.

2. Review the rationale for good nutrition.

3. Review the basic food groups.

4. Discuss current diet.

5. Discuss possible improvements in diet with the parent, if necessary.

    D. Rest and exercise
      1. Turn to this subsection of the health manual.
      2. Review each item and discuss them with parent when necessary.
    E. Regular medical checkups
      1. Turn to this subsection of the health manual.
      2. Review the schedule with the parent.
      3. Discuss strategies for maintaining this schedule.
    F. Immunization schedule.
      1. Turn to this subsection of the health manual.
      2. Review the schedule with the parent.
      3. Discuss strategies for maintaining this schedule.
IX. End the session
      1. Provide feedback to the parent regarding her or his performance during the session (descriptive praise and suggestions for improvement).
      2. Ask the parent to complete tasks before the next session.
        a. Complete planning forms.
        b. Get health supplies.
        c. Read Section 3 of the health manual, "Caring for Your Child at Home." Tell the parent this section includes material you will be covering in the next session.

Session 3

    I. Conduct a role-play scenario to assess parent performance. If parent has not yet scored 80% or better on a true–false quiz, administer a new true–false quiz. Administer a novel treat-at-home role-play scenario before beginning the training session.
   II. Provide performance feedback to parent.
      A. Provide positive and descriptive praise.
      B. Briefly review the steps missed.
      C. Have the parent practice the missed steps.
      D. Give feedback on practice.
  III. Make sure parent has the health manual and extra Parent Behavior Checklists and Health Recording Charts.
  IV. Describe the rationale for Training Session 3 (same as previous sessions).
   V. Briefly review the material covered in the previous session and answer any questions.
  VI. Review Section 3 of the manual, "Caring for Your Child at Home"
      A. Direct the parent to the appropriate section in the manual.
      B. Ask if she or he has had a chance to read it before the session.
      C. If the parent has read the material, answer any questions the parent may have. Ask if she or he would like to read it again together to make sure the material is clearly understood. If so, then read it again with her or him.
      D. If the parent has not read the material, read the section aloud with the parent and ask for and answer any questions.

VII. Provide the parent with feedback regarding her or his performance with the reading materials.

VIII. *Instructions, modeling, practice, and feedback.* Each skill should be discussed and modeled in its entirety for the parent. The parent should then be asked to practice the skill (either with a doll or with the child, when appropriate). Feedback should then be provided. Ask the parent to continue to practice steps not completed correctly, and provide assistance as necessary until the parent demonstrates the skills correctly.

A. Taking a pulse
1. Turn to this subsection of the health manual.
2. Review the three ways to take a pulse.
3. Select the method the parent is most likely to use (depending on the age of the child).
4. Demonstrate the skill for the parent (either on yourself or the child).
5. Ask the parent to show you how she or he would take the child's pulse.
6. Ask if she or he has felt the pulse.
7. Give positive feedback, and ask parent to repeat the skill until it is performed correctly.

B. Taking a temperature
1. Turn to this subsection of the health manual.
2. Review the four ways of taking a temperature (mercury, digital, armpit, and rectal).
3. Select the method the parent is most likely to use (depending on age of child and preference).
4. Demonstrate the skill for the parent (use a doll when necessary).
5. Tell the parent to show you how she or he would perform the skill.
6. Give positive feedback and, if necessary, ask the parent to continue to practice until the skill is performed correctly.
7. Discuss the tips for taking a temperature.

C. Giving medicine
1. Turn to this subsection of the health manual.
2. Review the four ways to give liquid medicine to a child.
3. Choose the method the parent is most likely to use.
4. Demonstrate that method (use water or juice if demonstrating with a child, *not* medicine).
5. Ask the parent to show you how she or he would give medicine using this method.
6. Give positive feedback, and if necessary, ask the parent to continue to practice until the skill is performed correctly.
7. Discuss additional tips for giving medications.

D. Giving drop medication
1. Turn to this subsection of the health manual.
2. Review the three types of drop medications (ear, nose, and eye).
3. Demonstrate how to administer each type.
4. Ask the parent to show you how she or he would administer each type.

5. Give positive feedback and, if necessary, ask parent to continue to practice until the skill is performed correctly.
6. Review tips for giving drop medicines.

E. Nursing a sick child
1. Turn to this subsection of the health manual.
2. Review the kinds of behavior that sick children sometimes demonstrate (crying, clinging, more demanding of attention, withdrawal).
3. Review appropriate parent responses (remaining calm and cheerful, being less demanding and more patient).
4. Review general tips for caring for sick children.
5. Answer any questions the parent has.

F. Comforting your child and activities for sick children
1. Turn to this subsection of the health manual.
2. Discuss the tips provided in the manual.
3. Discuss with the parent how she or he might use these tips.
4. Answer any questions the parent has.

G. Review the symptom and illness guide. Although the parent has already been introduced to this through the role-play scenarios, this is a more in-depth review of the symptom guide.
1. Turn to the symptom and illness guide.
2. Discuss and demonstrate how this section is used.
3. Review the symptoms that are included in this section by reading over the table of contents. Point out that symptoms are listed alphabetically.
4. Ask if the parent has used the guide in any real health-care situations yet. If so, ask how it went, and praise efforts to incorporate newly learned skills into real-life situations.
5. Point out that the parent does not need to memorize the guide but should be familiar enough with it to quickly refer to the appropriate information that is needed when the child becomes ill.

IX. End the session
A. Provide feedback to the parent regarding performance during the session (descriptive praise and suggestions for improvement).
B. Ask the parent to complete the following tasks before the next session.
1. Any remaining tasks from previous sessions (complete planning forms, get health supplies)
2. Read Sections 4 and 5 of the health manual, Calling the Doctor and Urgent Care. Tell her or him that these sections include material you will be covering in the next session.

Session 4

I. Conduct a role-play scenario to assess parent performance. If parent has not yet scored 80% or better on a true–false quiz, administer a new quiz. Administer a novel treat-at-home role-play scenario before beginning the training session.

II. Provide performance feedback to parent.
  A. Provide positive and descriptive praise.
  B. Briefly review the steps missed.
  C. Ask parent to practice the missed steps.
  D. Give feedback on practice.
III. Make sure parent has the health manual and extra Parent Behavior Checklists and Health Recording Charts.
IV. Describe the rationale for Training Session 4 (same as previous sessions, in addition to learning how to recognize when to call the doctor or to seek emergency treatment and how to go about these steps).
V. Briefly review the material covered in the previous session and answer any questions.
VI. Review Sections 4 and 5 of the manual, "Calling the Doctor" and "Urgent Care."
  A. Direct the parent to the appropriate sections in the manual.
  B. Ask if she or he has had a chance to read them before the session.
  C. If the parent has read the material, answer any questions the parent may have. Ask if she or he would like to read it again together to make sure the material is clearly understood. If so, then read it again with her or him.
  D. If the parent has not read the material, read the section aloud with the parent and ask for and answer any questions.
VII. Provide the parent with feedback regarding her or his performance with the reading materials.
VIII. *Instructions, modeling, practice, and feedback.* Each skill should be discussed and modeled in its entirety for the parent. The parent should then be asked to practice the skill (either with a doll or with the child, when appropriate). Feedback should then be provided. Ask the parent to continue to practice steps not completed correctly and provide assistance as necessary until the parent demonstrates the skills correctly.
  A. Calling the doctor (the term "doctor" is used during discussions with parents, who are likely to use this term rather than "physician").
    1. Turn to this section of the health manual.
    2. Briefly review the conditions under which to call the doctor.
    3. Review using the Health Recording Chart.
      a. Information to tell the doctor.
      b. What the parent should expect from the doctor.
      c. Why and how to record the doctor's instructions.
    4. Model calling the doctor using a novel "call the doctor" role-play scenario. Demonstrate all of the steps.
    5. Ask the parent to practice all of the steps for calling the doctor, using a novel role-play scenario.
    6. Provide positive feedback and, if necessary, ask the parent to continue practicing until all steps are completed correctly.
  B. Urgent care
    1. Turn to this section of the health manual.
    2. Briefly review ways to seek emergency treatment.

3. Briefly review conditions under which to seek emergency treatment.
4. Model seeking emergency treatment using a novel "emergency treatment" role-play scenario.
5. Ask the parent to practice all of the steps for seeking urgent care using a novel "emergency treatment" role-play scenario.
6. Provide positive feedback and, if necessary, ask the parent to continue practicing until all steps are completed correctly.
7. Briefly review first-aid procedures.

IX. End the session
   A. Provide feedback to the parent regarding performance during the session (descriptive praise and suggestions for improvement).
   B. Ask the parent to complete the following tasks before the next session.
      1. Any remaining tasks from previous sessions (complete planning forms, get health supplies).
      2. Use these skills whenever your child is ill.
      3. Be sure to use the recording sheets.
   C. Explain that the next session will consist of a number of opportunities to demonstrate that the parent has mastered the material. This session may be slightly longer than previous sessions if the parent does not score 100% on the scenarios right away; but if a little extra time is allowed for practice, this will be the final health session. If she or he has any difficulties, however, you will schedule one more practice session.

Session 5

I. You should have already prepared the following in advance:
   A. Three "treat at home" scenarios
   B. Three "call the doctor" scenarios
   C. Three "treat at home, then call the doctor" scenarios
   D. Three "emergency treatment" scenarios
   (*Note: At this point, some of the scenarios may not be novel to the parent. Although there is no prescribed order in which scenarios should be implemented throughout training, you can begin with the scenarios first introduced during assessment and the early training sessions. Also, the "treat at home, then call the doctor" scenarios are optional here because parents will be practicing "treat-at home" and "call the doctor" scenarios to criterion.*)

II. Describe the rationale for this session. The purpose of this session is to review all materials and to provide any additional practice the parent may need in order to complete each type of role-play scenario correctly (i.e., treat at home, call the doctor, and emergency treatment). If the parent has mastered the material, the session will be short. If the parent has trouble, then the session may be relatively long. An additional session may be scheduled to provide additional opportunities to practice, rather than allowing the session to last too long for the parent. Use best judgment in this case.

III. "Treat at home" scenarios.
   A. Administer a novel scenario (see preceding Note).
   B. If parent performed 100% of steps correctly, give positive and descriptive praise.
   C. If parent missed any steps:
      1. Review steps missed.
      2. Ask parent to practice the missed steps.
   D. Repeat with a different treat-at-home scenario until parent performs at 100% mastery criterion or until she or he has completed three role plays.

IV. "Call the doctor" scenarios
   A. Administer a novel scenario (see preceding Note).
   B. If parent performed 100% of steps correctly, give positive and descriptive praise.
   C. If parent missed any steps:
      1. Review steps missed.
      2. Ask parent to practice the missed steps.
   D. Repeat with a different call-the-doctor scenario until parent performs at 100% mastery criterion or until she or he has completed three role plays.
      (*Note: You may use "Treat at home, then call the doctor" scenario in place of one treat-at-home scenario and one call-the-doctor scenario.*)

V. "Emergency treatment" scenario
   A. Administer a novel scenario.
   B. If parent performed 100% of steps correctly, give positive and descriptive praise.
   C. If parent missed any steps:
      1. Review steps missed.
      2. Ask parent to practice the missed steps.
   D. Repeat with a different emergency-treatment scenario until parent performs at 100% mastery criterion or until she or he has completed two role plays.

VI. Determine if an additional session should be scheduled.
   A. If the parent performed 100% of the steps correctly for each of the categories of scenarios, then she or he has met the mastery criterion, and an additional session is unnecessary. Provide praise for successfully completing the training package.
   B. If the parent did not score 100% correct at least once within any one of the categories of scenarios, then an additional session should be scheduled. Reassure the parent that many parents require an extra session to master all of the skills necessary for dealing with such a broad range of illnesses.

VII. Review the session.
   A. Briefly review the material covered during training by referring to the table of contents in the health manual and the symptom and illness guide.
   B. Answer any questions the parent may have.

VIII. End the session.
   A. Give parent positive and descriptive feedback about performance during the session and throughout the training.
   B. Encourage the parent to continue to use the skills.
   C. Prompt the parent to keep the materials in a safe place and to continue to use them.

FOLLOW-UP SESSIONS

Follow-up observations should be conducted up to 6 months following the completion of training, but they can be conducted more frequently. During each observation, the counselor conducts one treat-at-home, one call-the-doctor, or one treat-at-home-then-call-the-doctor combination role-play scenario and one emergency-treatment scenario. A true–false quiz is also administered. Follow-up sessions provide an opportunity to assess maintenance of parents' health care skills over time. They also can be informative in determining whether booster-training sessions are needed.

CONSUMER SATISFACTION SURVEY

Following the final training session, a consumer satisfaction questionnaire (see Appendix 7.10) is presented to each family with the request to rate the usefulness of the training procedures, their satisfaction with the counselor's performance, and whether they would recommend this training program to other parents. This questionnaire provides an additional opportunity for parents to provide feedback to the counselors regarding the relevance of the training package and the way in which it was implemented.

COMMON PROBLEMS AND SOLUTIONS

In some cases, parents may be uncomfortable role playing health care skills. As discussed in Chapter 5, a counselor should both fully explain the importance of role playing to developing new skills and offer to role play for the parent in some scenarios. Another problem that is frequently observed while conducting health training is due to cultural differences. In some cases, families of different cultures have different views about health care and may resort to folk remedies when family members are ill. In these cases, it is important to individually evaluate the parents' practices. It is important to balance the essential need to ensure that children receive adequate health care with your attempts to work with the parents within their culture. Consulting the appropriate health professional who has experience with a given cultural group may provide some background about the family's practices and offer some solutions to dealing with these differences.

Finally, because of financial limitations, it may be difficult for some families to obtain the necessary medical supplies, such as bandages, acetaminophen, or a thermometer. In Project SafeCare, families were provided with a set of medical supplies. If you are unable to provide these supplies, contact local companies who may have the resources to provide a donation or discount. Further, it would be helpful to be aware of free or low-cost clinics in local neighborhoods that could provide health care to families.

CASE EXAMPLES

Maria, a mother of five children, was referred to Project SafeCare because of reports of neglect. After training, she used her health manual, symptom guide, and Health Recording Chart when her son became ill. The youngest of her children, Adam, complained of feeling sick, and after feeling her son's forehead, Maria found that he felt warm. Maria asked her son further questions to determine what the problem was and discovered that her child had an earache. Maria determined that the likely cause of her child's illness was an ear infection accompanied by a slight fever. After recording her son's symptoms on the Health Recording Chart and consulting the symptom guide, the mother called the physician as directed. The nurse told her to come into the physician's office. The physician then prescribed antibiotics and children's acetaminophen, which, given for the prescribed amount of time, resulted in successful treatment of the ear infection. In addition to following instructions to call the physician, Maria tried the suggestions described in the symptom guide to make her son more comfortable. These tips included placing a hot water bottle covered with a towel next to her child's ear to relieve pain and protecting the ear from water during bath time. Maria recorded all of these steps, including the time and dosage of each administration of medication she gave to her son, on her Health Recording Chart.

Another parent, Julia, a single teenage mother with a newborn infant, reported that her son, Jorge, developed diaper rash shortly after she completed training. On noticing the symptoms, she recorded them on her Health Recording Chart and referred to her symptom guide. The section on diaper rash directed her to spread a diaper cream on the affected area, to wash her child's bottom after each bowel movement, and to allow her son to lie on a blanket without a diaper when possible. Julia reported that the diaper rash cleared up within a couple of days and that she would definitely use her health manual and symptom guide and the Health Recording Charts whenever Jorge developed similar symptoms or became ill in the future.

Sample True–False Quiz

Name _____   Date _____

Circle one: Baseline   Treatment   Follow-up

For each statement below, circle T for True or F for False.

T   F   1. A diaper should be changed as soon as it becomes wet or soiled to reduce the likelihood of diaper rash.

T   F   2. If your child has diarrhea, you should not give him or her any fluids so that the stools become less runny.

T   F   3. If your child's forehead feels hot, there is nothing to worry about; you don't need to take his or her temperature unless he or she complains of pain.

T   F   4. If your child complains of a sore ear or your infant cries and pulls at her or his ear, you don't need to do anything about it; this is normal with an earache.

T   F   5. If you are not sure how much medicine to give to your child, you should call the doctor for advice.

T   F   6. When your child has a fever, only solid foods and no liquids should be given to him or her.

T   F   7. When you give liquid medicine to an infant, you should pour it all into the infant's mouth at once so that he or she does not have time to spit any out.

T   F   8. Baby formula can be prepared however you think your baby likes it best without worrying about the instructions on the container.

T   F   9. It is important to bring your child to the doctor for regular checkups even when your child is well.

T   F   10. If your child is congested, it may help to run hot water in the shower to make the bathroom steamy, and then bring your child into the bathroom and let him or her breathe in the steam.

(answers: 1. True; 2. False; 3. False; 4. False; 5. True; 6. False; 7. False; 8. False; 9. True; 10. True)

Symptoms Depicted in the Set of Scenario Cards

Scenario	Illness depicted	Correct treatment
1	Cold	Treat at home
2	Chicken pox	Call the doctor
3	Diaper Rash	Treat at home, then call the doctor
4	Convulsion	Emergency treatment
5	Fever (child under 6 months)	Call the doctor
6	Cough	Treat at home
7	Stomachache	Treat at home
8	Constipation	Call the doctor
9	Measles	Call the doctor
10	Earache	Call the doctor
11	Stomachache with vomiting	Treat at home, then call the doctor
12	Diaper Rash	Treat at home
13	Diarrhea	Treat at home
14	Fever	Treat at home, then call the doctor
15	Vomiting	Call the doctor
16	Chicken pox (already diagnosed)	Treat at home
17	Broken leg/limping	Emergency treatment
18	Vomiting (4-month-old child)	Emergency treatment
19	Dehydration	Emergency treatment

Sample Scenario Cards

Scenario 1

When changing your baby's diaper, you notice redness around his thighs, bottom, and genital area. The skin feels moist, and he cries when you touch him there. His skin looks tight and shiny, and you also notice a strong smell of ammonia. Tell the counselor what you think the problem is and show him or her what you would do.

Scenario 2

Your child is 5 years old and has red spots on her face, neck, chest, and stomach. She is scratching the spots all the time and complaining that she is uncomfortable. When you took her temperature, you discovered that she had a slight fever (100.8°F or 38°C). Please tell the counselor what you think the problem is and show him or her what you would do.

Scenario 3

Your child has been crying a lot. She is refusing to eat her breakfast. Last night she vomited twice, and she had a hard time falling asleep. She has been holding her stomach and complaining that it hurts. Tell the counselor what you think the problem is and show him or her what you would do.

Scenario 4

Your 8-month-old has had diarrhea for 1½ days. She does not seem to want to eat or drink. Her mouth and lips are dry, and her urine is very dark yellow. She also does not seem to have any energy. Tell the counselor what you think the problem is and show him or her what you would do.

Sample Scenario Answer Sheet

Scenario 1 (Treat at home)   **Diaper Rash**

When changing your baby's diaper, you notice redness around his thighs, bottom, and genital area. The skin feels moist, and he cries when you touch him there. His skin looks tight and shiny, and you also notice a strong smell of ammonia. Tell the counselor what you think the problem is and show him or her what you would do.

SYMPTOMS
Acceptable: diaper rash, rash, sore bottom Unacceptable: sick, something wrong, smells bad

CORRECT RESPONSE: TREAT AT HOME

Check Symptoms		Treatment	
Temp.	Other	Acceptable	Unacceptable
1. 98.6°F 2. 98.6°F 3. 98.6°F	1. Rash and tender thighs and bottom; crying 2. *Rash, less tender/ same as 1 3. *Less rash, not tender/ same as 1	• **Wash bottom with warm water.** • **Apply diaper rash ointment or petroleum jelly.** • **Change diapers and wash bottom every 2–3 hours** • Leave diaper off when possible • Check inside of mouth for thrush • Change diaper brand	• Talcum powder on rash • Baking soda on rash • Use plastic pants

* If symptoms were treated correctly when checked, give the response before the "/." If symptoms were *not* treated correctly, give the response after the "/."

Bold items are essential steps. Unbolded items are helpful, but these responses are not required.

INCORRECT RESPONSE

If parent says she or he would call the doctor:
   • Ask for symptoms if parent does not give them.
   • Recommend leaving child's diaper off, washing area frequently, and applying Desitin lotion. If not better in 2 days, call back.
 	
If parent says she or he would take the child to the emergency room:
   • End the role play.
 	
If this scenario is conducted during training, after scenario is over tell parent that she or he should have treated at home. Discuss the correct steps.

(continued)

Scenario 2 (Call the doctor)   **Chicken Pox**

Your child is 5 years old and has red spots on her face, neck, chest, and stomach. She is scratching the spots all the time and complaining that she is uncomfortable. When you took her temperature, you discovered that she had a slight fever (100.8°F or 38°C). Please tell the counselor what you think the problem is and show him or her what you would do.

SYMPTOMS

Acceptable: chicken pox, rash, fever and rash
Unacceptable: sick, whining

CORRECT RESPONSE: CALL THE DOCTOR

Check Symptoms		Treatment
Temp.	Other	Call Doctor
1. 100.8°F	1. Intense itchiness, small blisters, fever	• Ask for symptoms if parent does not give them.
2. 98.6°F/ 100.9°F	2. Small blisters, itching	• Tell parent to bring child in to make sure it is chicken pox.
3. 98.6°F/ 100.8°F	3. Small blisters, itching	• Schedule appointment.
		• End role play.

* If symptoms were treated correctly when checked, give the response before the "/." If symptoms were *not* treated correctly, give the response after the "/."

INCORRECT RESPONSE

If parent says she or he would treat at home:
  • Use the symptoms listed under "check symptoms" to play along.

If parent says she would take the child to the emergency room:
  • End the role play.

If this scenario is conducted during training, after scenario is over tell parent that she or he should have consulted the doctor.

(continued)

Scenario 3 (Treat at home, then call the doctor) **Stomachache with Vomiting**

Your child has been crying a lot. She is refusing to eat her breakfast. Last night she vomited twice, and she had a hard time falling asleep. She has been holding her stomach and complaining that it hurts. Tell the counselor what you think the problem is and show him or her what you would do.

SYMPTOMS

Acceptable: vomiting, stomachache
Unacceptable: sick, in pain

CORRECT RESPONSE: TREAT AT HOME, THEN CALL THE DOCTOR

Check Symptoms	
Temp.	Other
1. 98.6°F	1. Vomiting, not eating
2. 100.8°F	2. Same as #1, plus diarrhea
3. 102.0°F	3. After 24 hours, same as #2

Treatment	
Acceptable	Unacceptable
• **Clear liquids only**	• Any medication
• Put child to bed	• Keeping child on a regular diet.
• **At Step #2, call the doctor.**	

Call Doctor
• **Ask for symptoms if parent does not give them.**
• **Tell parent to come in right away.**

Bold items are essential steps. Unbolded items are helpful, but these responses are not required.

INCORRECT RESPONSE

If parent says she or he would call the doctor at Step #1:
• Role play call to the doctor. Although the parent should wait for the second symptom check to call the doctor, as long as the parent calls the doctor, this can be considered correct.

If parent treats at home without calling the doctor:
• If the parent does not call the doctor after 24 hours, end the role play.

If the parent chooses emergency treatment:
• End the role play.

If this scenario is conducted during training, after scenario is over tell parent that she or he should have watched the symptoms for a little while, tried to treat at home with clear liquids, and with the next symptom check (temperature increased and diarrhea appeared), she or he should have called the doctor. Role play steps involved in calling the doctor.

(continued)

Scenario 4 (Emergency Treatment)   **Dehydration**

Your 8-month-old has had diarrhea for 1½ days. She does not seem to want to eat or drink. Her mouth and lips are dry, and her urine is very dark yellow. She also does not seem to have any energy. Tell the counselor what you think the problem is and show him or her what you would do.

SYMPTOMS
Acceptable: dehydration, diarrhea, dry mouth Unacceptable: sick, lethargic, not hungry, lazy

CORRECT RESPONSE: SEEK EMERGENCY TREATMENT

Check Symptoms	
Temp	Other
1. 100.0°F	1. Diarrhea, dry mouth, not eating, no energy, concentrated urine
2. 102.0°F	2. Same as #1, plus not urinating for 4 hours
3. 102.0°F	3. Same as #2, plus soft spot on head sunken in

INCORRECT RESPONSE
If parent says she or he would treat at home: • Use the symptoms listed under "check symptoms" to play along. If parent says she or he would call the doctor: • Role-play the call to the doctor. • Ask for symptoms if parent does not give them. • Advise parent to bring the child to the emergency room or call 911 immediately. If this scenario is conducted during training, after scenario is over inform parent that she or he should have sought emergency treatment right away.

Symptoms and Illnesses Discussed
in the Health Symptom and Illness Guide

Abdominal pain

Appetite loss

Bronchitis

Chicken pox

Cold

Colic

Constipation

Convulsions

Cough

Cradle cap

Croup

Crying

Dehydration

Diaper rash

Diarrhea

Earache

Failure to thrive

Feeding problems

Fever

German measles (rubella)

Headache

Influenza (flu)

Itching

Jaundice

Limping

Measles

Mumps

Rash

Seizures

Sleep problems

Sore throat

Stomachache

Swelling

Teething

Vomiting

Parent Behavior Checklist—Counselor's Version

Parent: _____

Observer: _____ (P R)

Condition: Bl   Trtmt   Follow-up

Key: +   correct

      –   incorrect

N/A not applicable

Date:

Scenario Card Number:

A. General Steps
  1. States problem
  2. Records symptoms on recording chart
  3. Checks the health manual and finds symptoms or possible illnesses

B. Call the Doctor
  1. Recording chart ready
  2. Pencil
  3. Child nearby
  4. Describes symptoms
  5. Records instructions
  6. Follows physician's instructions

C. Seek Emergency Treatment

D. Treat at Home
  1. Gets recommended supplies from medicine cabinet
  2. Reads instructions on medication label or in reference book
  3. Follows instructions for administering treatment
  4. Records treatment on recording chart

  5. Checks again and states symptoms present after length of time recommended by reference book
  6. Records symptoms on recording chart
  7. If symptoms still present, calls physician or readministers treatment, as recommended
  8. Records treatment on recording chart

  9. Checks again and states symptoms present at the time recommended by reference book
  10. Records symptoms on recording chart
  11. If symptoms still present, calls physician or readministers treatment as recommended
  12. Records treatment on recording chart
  13. If symptoms are gone, stops treatment unless otherwise instructed by physician, health care professional, or reference book

Total steps correct

Total steps correct (+) and incorrect (–)

Percent correct

Total agreement

Parent Behavior Checklist—Parent's Version

A. General Steps

Regardless of the appropriate treatment, always follow these general steps:

- ☐ Identify your child's symptoms
- ☐ Record the symptoms on the Health Recording Chart
- ☐ Look for symptoms or illness in the Health Manual
- ☐ Determine if you need to . . .
    - ☐ Seek emergency treatment
    - ☐ Call the doctor
    - ☐ Treat at home

B. Call the Doctor

If you need to call the doctor, follow these steps:

- ☐ Have Health Recording Chart ready
- ☐ Have a pencil or pen ready
- ☐ Have your child nearby
- ☐ Describe the symptoms to the doctor
- ☐ Write down what the doctor tells you
- ☐ Follow the doctor's instructions

C. Treat at Home

If you can treat the symptoms at home, follow these steps:

- ☐ Get recommended items (from medicine cabinet or other)
- ☐ Read instructions for all medicine before giving to child
- ☐ Follow instructions for giving medicine to child
- ☐ Write time, medicine, and dose on Health Recording Chart
- ☐ Check symptoms again after recommended time
- ☐ Write symptoms on Health Recording Chart
- ☐ If symptoms still present, treat illness or call doctor
- ☐ Record treatment on Health Recording Chart
- ☐ Check symptoms again after recommended time
- ☐ Write symptoms on Health Recording Chart
- ☐ If symptoms still present, treat illness or call doctor
- ☐ Record treatment on Health Recording Chart
- ☐ If symptoms gone, stop treatment unless otherwise instructed
- ☐ Continue until child is better

Operational Definitions and Scoring Guidelines for the Parent Behavior Checklist

A. General Steps

1. *States problem.* The parent says what symptoms are present on the scenario card. Parent does not have to repeat all symptoms verbatim but should identify the primary symptom or name an illness that would have similar symptoms. If what the parent describes would be enough to lead to a probable diagnosis or an appropriate course of action using the health manual or another reference material, then it is considered a sufficient description of the problem. The scenario card answer sheet will indicate acceptable and unacceptable responses.

   Example: Scenario card indicates that a child feels warm, is cranky, and has loose stools.

   Acceptable Responses (+): Child has diarrhea, child might have diarrhea and a fever; child has runny stools.

   Unacceptable Responses (–): Child is sick, child doesn't feel well, child needs to go to the doctor.

2. *Records symptoms on the Health Recording Chart.* The parent writes the symptoms described in the scenario onto the Health Recording Chart (after having received the health manual), *or* the parent writes the symptoms on a piece of paper or in a notebook.

   Example: Scenario card indicates that a child feels warm, is cranky, and has loose stools.

   Acceptable Responses (+): Parent takes out a copy of the Health Recording Chart and writes the symptoms (warm, cranky, loose stools) in the appropriate space on the chart; parent writes the symptoms on a piece of paper or in a notebook.

   Unacceptable Responses (–): Parent does not write any symptoms on any paper.

3. *Checks the health manual and finds symptoms or possible illnesses.* The parent gets the health manual or another reference book or materials that contain information about children's illnesses.

   Example: Scenario card indicates that a child feels warm, is cranky, and has loose stools.

   Acceptable Responses (+): Parent gets the health manual and looks up loose stools, parent reads description of loose stools, including possible illnesses. Parent gets appropriate reference material and looks up loose stools; reads description of loose stools, including possible illnesses. Parent gets health manual and looks up diarrhea. Parent gets appropriate reference material and looks up diarrhea; Parent asks another person (friend or relative) to help her or him read or read to her or him the description of loose stools.

   Unacceptable Responses (–): Parent does not refer to any reference material; parent says she or he does not know what to do; parent calls doctor or emergency room.

   (continued)

Note: Refer to the scenario card answer sheet to determine if the scenario requires a parent to call a health care professional, to seek emergency treatment, or to treat at home. Then score only the section that applies for the scenario. This will be indicated on the scenario card answer sheet.

B. Call the Doctor

1. *Recording chart ready*. Parent has a copy of a Health Recording Chart or other paper or notebook in which symptoms are written.

    Acceptable Responses (+): Parent gets the Health Recording Chart and holds it or places it near the telephone.

    Unacceptable Responses (–): Parent has no paper or recording chart available.

2. *Pencil*.

    Acceptable Responses (+): Parent gets a pen or pencil and holds it or places it near the phone.

    Unacceptable Responses (–): Parent does not have a pen or pencil available.

3. *Child nearby*. Parent brings the child to the telephone so that the child will be available in case the doctor asks the parent to check for any additional symptoms.

    Acceptable Responses (+): Parent asks the child to sit or stand near the telephone; parent holds small child; parent has doll nearby (if using a doll rather than child in role play).

    Unacceptable Responses (–): Child is left in another room; small child (i.e., one who does not walk independently) is in same room but out of parent's reach.

4. *Describes symptoms*. Parent describes symptoms to the health care professional.

    Acceptable Responses (+): Child has diarrhea; child might have diarrhea and fever; child has runny stools.

    Unacceptable Responses (–): Child is sick; child does not feel well, child needs to go to doctor.

5. *Records instructions*. Using the Health Recording Chart, a piece of paper, or a notepad, parent accurately writes down the instructions she receives from the health care professional.

    Acceptable Responses (+): Parent writes instructions onto Health Recording Chart, a piece of paper, or a notepad. Parent's notes must be accurate.

    Unacceptable Responses (–): Parent does not write down the instructions given by the health care professional; parent writes down inaccurate instructions.

    Note: The scenario card answer sheet provides the information the counselor needs in order to role play the part of the health care professional.

(continued)

6. *Follows physician's instructions.* Parent does what the health care professional tells her or him to do.

Acceptable Responses (+): The acceptable response depends on the advice of the health care professional and will be one of the following: (1) parent will go to the emergency room; (2) parent makes an appointment with doctor; or (3) parent completes the treat-at-home steps as advised by the doctor.

Unacceptable Responses (–): Parent does nothing; parent engages in some other behavior that was not recommended by the doctor (e.g., doctor says to treat at home but parent says she or he would go to the emergency room).

Note. If parent has been instructed by the health care professional to treat at home, score only step B6; *do not* score treat-at-home steps.

C. Seek Emergency Treatment

Acceptable Responses (+): Parent says she would go to the emergency room; parent says she would call 911 or an ambulance.

Unacceptable Responses (–): Parent calls health care professional; parent treats at home; parent does nothing.

D. Treat at Home

1. *Gets recommended supplies from medicine cabinet.*

Acceptable Responses (+): Parent goes to medicine cabinet or other area in which medical supplies are kept and gets the items recommended by the health care professional or in the health manual or other appropriate reference material.

Unacceptable Responses (–): Parent does not get any medical supplies; parent gets medical supplies that were not recommended by the health care professional, health manual, or other appropriate reference material.

Not Applicable (N/A): The health manual, reference materials, and/or doctor recommend a treatment that does not require any medical supplies.

2. *Reads instructions on medication label or in reference book.*

Acceptable Responses (+): Parent looks at the label on the medicine container or at the section of the reference material that provides instructions about how to administer treatment.

Unacceptable Response (–): Parent does not look at label or at appropriate section of reference materials.

Not Applicable (N/A): The health manual, reference materials, and/or doctor do not recommend a medicine or treatment.

(continued)

3. *Follows instructions for administering treatment.*

   Acceptable Responses (+): Parent administers the medicine or the treatment appropriately (i.e., according to the written instructions on the label or in the reference material). *Note.* Parent does not have to be looking at instructions while administering medicine or treatment. This step is independent of performance on step D2.

   Unacceptable Responses (−): Parent does not administer medicine or treatment when one is recommended; parent does not administer medicine or treatment correctly (i.e., according to written instructions on label or in reference materials).

   Note. If label and reference materials give conflicting instructions, use instructions on label as guide.

   Not Applicable (N/A): The health manual, reference materials, and/or doctor do not recommend a medicine or treatment.

4. *Records treatment on recording chart.*

   Acceptable Responses (+): On the Health Recording Chart *or* on a piece of paper or notepad, the parent writes down the name and amount of medicine administered and the time of administration and/or a description of the treatment administered and the time of administration.

   Unacceptable Responses (−): Parent does not write down the name and amount of medicine administered or the time of administration and/or does not write down a description of the treatment administered or the time of administration.

   Not Applicable (N/A): The health manual, reference materials, and/or doctor do not recommend a medicine or treatment.

5. *Checks again and states symptoms present after length of the time recommended by reference book.*

   If parent states that she or he would check on symptoms again, ask when she or he would check, give her or him additional information from the scenario card answer sheet regarding symptoms at check time, and tell her or him to show you what she or he would do.

   If parent does not indicate intention to check on symptoms again, score this step as unacceptable (−), but give parent additional information from scenario card about child's symptoms at the check time and go on to the next step.

   Acceptable Responses (+): Parent states that she or he would check symptoms again at the time recommended by the health manual or other appropriate reference material or by doctor (e.g., after 2 hours, after 4 hours, etc.), and parent correctly states symptoms present (as in Step A1).

   Unacceptable Responses (−): Parent does not state intention to check on symptoms again; parent states intention to check on symptoms again but does not check at the time

(continued)

recommended by the health manual or other appropriate reference materials; parent states intention to check at the recommended time but misidentifies the symptoms or does not state the symptoms (see Step A1).

Note. The scenario card answer sheet provides the information needed to tell the parent about symptoms for each opportunity to check.

6. *Records symptoms on recording chart.*

   Example: Scenario card instructs counselor to indicate that a child still feels warm and has loose stools.

   Acceptable Responses (+): Parent takes out a copy of the Health Recording Chart and accurately writes the symptoms (warm, loose bowels) in the appropriate space on the chart; parent writes the symptoms on a piece of paper or notepad.

   Unacceptable Responses (–): Parent does not write any symptoms on any paper.

   Not Applicable (N/A): Scenario card indicates that the child no longer has symptoms.

7. *If symptoms still present, calls physician or readministers treatment as recommended.*

   Acceptable Responses (+): Parent calls health care professional and/or parent readministers treatment, as recommended in health manual or other reference material.

   Unacceptable Responses (–): Parent does not call health care professional or readminister treatment when reference materials indicate to do so; parent calls health care professional when reference materials indicate that parent should readminister treatment, seek emergency treatment, or do nothing; parent readministers treatment when reference materials indicate parent should call health care professional, seek emergency treatment, or do nothing.

   Note. If parent needs to call health care professional, score this step, then begin scoring the steps for calling the doctor. Score Steps 8 to 13 as "not applicable." If parent does *not* call health care professional, score this step as incorrect (–) *and* score the steps for calling the doctor as incorrect (–).

8. *Records treatment on recording chart.*

   Acceptable Responses (+): On the Health Recording Chart *or* on a piece of paper or notepad, the parent writes down the name and amount of medicine administered and the time of administration and/or a description of the treatment administered and the time of administration.

   Unacceptable Responses (–): Parent does not write down the name and amount of medicine administered or the time of administration and/or does not write down a description of the treatment administered or the time of administration.

   Not Applicable (N/A): The health manual, reference materials, and/or doctor do not recommend a medicine or treatment.

(continued)

9. *Checks again and states symptoms present at the time recommended by reference book.*

If parent states intention to check on symptoms again, ask when she or he would check, give her or him additional information from the scenario card answer sheet regarding symptoms at check time, and tell her or him to show you what she or he would do.

If parent does not indicate intention to check on symptoms again, score this step as unacceptable (–), but give parent additional information from scenario card about child's symptoms at the check time and go on to the next step.

Acceptable Responses (+): Parent states that she or he would check symptoms again at the time recommended by the health manual or other appropriate reference material or by doctor (e.g., after 2 hours, after 4 hours, etc.), and parent correctly states symptoms present (as in Step A1).

Unacceptable Responses (–): Parent does not state intention to check on symptoms again; parent states intention to check on symptoms again but does not check at the time recommended by the health manual or other appropriate reference materials; parent states intention to check at the recommended time but misidentifies the symptoms or does not state the symptoms (see Step A1).

Note. The scenario card answer sheet provides the information needed to tell the parent about symptoms for each opportunity to check.

10. *Records symptoms on recording chart.*

Example: Scenario card instructs counselor to indicate that a child still feels warm and has loose stools.

Acceptable Responses (+): Parent takes out a copy of the Health Recording Chart and accurately writes the symptoms (warm; loose stools) in the appropriate space on the chart; parent writes the symptoms on a piece of paper or notepad.

Unacceptable Responses (–): Parent does not write any symptoms on any paper.

Not Applicable (N/A): Scenario card indicates that the child no longer has symptoms.

11. *If symptoms still present, calls physician or* readministers treatment as recommended.

Acceptable Responses (+): Parent calls health care professional and/or parent readministers treatment, as recommended in health manual or other reference material.

Unacceptable Responses (–): Parent does not call health care professional or readminister treatment when reference materials indicate to do so; parent calls health care professional when reference materials indicate that parent should readminister treatment, seek emergency treatment, or do nothing; parent readministers treatment when reference materials indicate parent should call health care professional, seek emergency treatment, or do nothing.

(continued)

Note. If parent needs to call health care professional, score this step, then begin scoring the steps for calling the doctor. Score Steps 8 to 13 as "not applicable." If parent does *not* call health care professional, score this step as incorrect (–) *and* score the steps for calling the doctor as incorrect (–).

12. *Records treatment on recording chart.*

   Acceptable Responses (+): On the Health Recording Chart *or* on a piece of paper or notepad, the parent writes down the name and amount of medicine administered and the time of administration and/or a description of the treatment administered and the time of administration.

   Unacceptable Responses (–): Parent does not write down the name and amount of medicine administered or the time of administration and/or does not write down a description of the treatment administered or the time of administration.

   Not Applicable (N/A): The health manual, reference materials, and/or doctor do not recommend a medicine or treatment.

13. *If symptoms are gone, stops treatment unless otherwise instructed by physician, health care professional, or reference book.*

   Acceptable Responses (+): Parent does not readminister treatment if symptoms are no longer present *and* treatment can be discontinued (according to health care professional or reference materials); parent readministers treatment according to instructions provided by health care professional or reference materials.

   Unacceptable Responses (–): Parent does not readminister treatment when health care professional or reference materials indicate that treatment should be readministered; parent readministers treatment in absence of symptoms when health care professional or reference materials have not indicated that treatment should be readministered or have indicated that treatment should not be readministered.

Scoring Instructions

Refer to the bottom of the counselor's version of the Parent Behavior Checklist (Appendix 7.6).

Total steps correct. Count the number of steps that received a correct (+) score and record in this box.

Total steps correct and incorrect. Count the total number of steps scored correct (+) *and* incorrect (–) and record in this box. Do not count the steps scored N/A or the steps not scored.

Percent correct: Divide the total steps correct (+) by the total steps and divide by 100. Record in this box.

Total agreement: Divide the total number of steps on which both observers agreed by the total number of steps scored and multiply by 100. Record this in the box.

$$\frac{\text{Agreements}}{\text{Agreements} + \text{Disagreements}} \times 100 = \text{Percent agreement}$$

Health Recording Chart

Date: _____

Child's name: _____
Age: _____ Approx. Weight: _____

Allergies to any medications?   Yes   No
If yes, list all medications: _____
_____
Other allergies: _____

Symptoms:

_____
_____
_____
_____
_____

Medicine/treatments given:

_____
_____
_____
_____
_____

Time checked	Symptoms still present?	Temperature?	Medicine/treatment readministered?	Call the doctor?
A.M. P.M.	Yes No	No Yes: _____	Yes No	Yes No
A.M. P.M.	Yes No	No Yes: _____	Yes No	Yes No
A.M. P.M.	Yes No	No Yes: _____	Yes No	Yes No
A.M. P.M.	Yes No	No Yes: _____	Yes No	Yes No

Call the Doctor: Doctor's name: _____   Phone number: _____

☐ Have pen and paper ready
☐ Have child nearby

List any illnesses the child has been exposed to recently: _____
_____

Be prepared to tell the doctor:
☐ Child's name and age   ☐ Child's symptoms (including temperature)
☐ Medicines/treatments given   ☐ Allergies

Record instructions from doctor: _____
_____
_____

Health Consumer Satisfaction Questionnaire

Thank you for participating in the health care training offered by Project SafeCare. We would like to learn some of your thoughts and feelings about the health training program. Information we receive from parents like you will be used to improve the program and its effectiveness. Please read the following comments and circle the answer that best describes your feelings about each statement. Be as honest as possible, as your responses will not affect your interactions with Project SafeCare or other agencies. A space has been provided for you to add additional comments. Thank you for your time and cooperation.

1. Caring for my child's health when he or she is ill has become easier.

Strongly agree	Agree	Neutral	Disagree	Strongly disagree
1	2	3	4	5

2. Recognizing that my child is ill has become easier.

Strongly agree	Agree	Neutral	Disagree	Strongly disagree
1	2	3	4	5

3. Knowing when to take my child to the doctor has become easier.

Strongly agree	Agree	Neutral	Disagree	Strongly disagree
1	2	3	4	5

4. It has become easier to recognize when my child needs emergency treatment.

Strongly agree	Agree	Neutral	Disagree	Strongly disagree
1	2	3	4	5

5. As a result of this program, I am more confident that I am better prepared to care for my child when he or she is sick.

Strongly agree	Agree	Neutral	Disagree	Strongly disagree
1	2	3	4	5

6. Buying medication and health supplies has become easier.

Strongly agree	Agree	Neutral	Disagree	Strongly disagree
1	2	3	4	5

7. When talking to my child's doctor, I feel more confident than before.

Strongly agree	Agree	Neutral	Disagree	Strongly disagree
1	2	3	4	5

(continued)

8. I believe that this health training program would be useful to other parents.

Strongly agree	Agree	Neutral	Disagree	Strongly disagree
1	2	3	4	5

9. I feel the health training program did <u>not</u> provide me with any new or useful information or skills.

Strongly agree	Agree	Neutral	Disagree	Strongly disagree
1	2	3	4	5

Rate how useful each of these items was in helping you benefit from the services you received, if relevant.

	Useful	Somewhat useful	OK	Slightly useful	Useless
1. Counselor's explanations					
2. Counselor's demonstrations					
3. Practice during sessions					
4. Practice outside of sessions					
5. Counselor's feedback					
6. Written materials					

Please rate the counselor who conducted the health training program.

	Strongly agree	Agree	Neutral	Disagree	Strongly disagree
1. Was warm and friendly					
2. Was helpful					
3. Gave clear explanations					
4. Was knowledgeable					
5. Was negative or critical					
6. Treated me fairly					
7. Was willing to spend extra time when I needed it					
8. Kept our scheduled appointments					
9. Was on time to scheduled appointments					
10. Interacted well with my child					

Comments:

8

Staff Training

SELECTION OF STAFF

Selection of staff is an important consideration in delivering the services described in this book. Different states, communities, and programs may have specific funding situations or requirements that make selection in terms of particular prerequisites necessary. Our own program has been university based, although our Project SafeCare data suggest that nurses, caseworkers, and graduate assistants, as well as use of video, are all at least mostly successful as the mediators of these services. It may be that parents who have successfully completed these protocols could serve as trainers also.

Our own preference for using graduate assistants to deliver these services is due to their being cost effective and not approaching burnout. Graduate assistants are still quite "fresh" and happy to be "doing good." We are able to pay them a decent salary, although salaries are not as high as and benefits are fewer than those of mental health professionals. Again, this does not preclude this prototype from being employed in such mental health settings; in fact, it has been. Graduate assistants are also motivated by other needs, such as practicum and internship credits, material for theses and dissertations, experience, and letters of recommendation.

The disadvantage of using graduate assistants is their youth, their part-time status (also an advantage because of the burnout factor), and their need for academic vacations. These factors can be largely overcome by the training we describe below. The training that we describe applies to all staff, whatever their credentials.

A PROTOTYPE FOR STAFF TRAINING

This volume serves as a "head start" for staff training in that we always begin with written materials, and we have provided them here. Our research and experience shows, however, that reading materials, whether they are intended for parents or staff, only serve to inform, not to train skills. Written materials should be used only as ancillary materials in training parents or staff. These materials never replace hands-on training.

The use of written materials requires a means of determining that the material they contain has been accurately and effectively presented; thus the trainee must pass quizzes to a set criterion. That is, the trainee should be able to pass the quiz by scoring at least 90% on objective test items and by meeting the full requirements of any short-answer or essay questions. We have included counselor training quizzes for the parent–child interaction, home safety and cleanliness, and health training components (see Appendices 8.1–8.3).

If a trainee fails a quiz, that is, scores below the 90% criterion, a supervisor reviews the missed items, asks the staff member to read the section of the training materials that pertains to the missed items, and, when ready, the trainee takes another version of the quiz. This practice is repeated until the trainee meets the criterion.

Modeling is another key component of staff training. Here, key skills of the particular training protocol are broken into discrete steps. During a behavioral simulation, the supervisor models each step of the training protocol. For example, the trainee may play the role of the parent in a role play or observe the supervisor role playing with another counselor. She or he observes the supervisor modeling an entire training session. The supervisor should be sure to demonstrate each step correctly. After the supervisor completes the role play, the counselor is then given an opportunity to practice the protocol. During this role play, the supervisor checks off each correctly completed step on the Counselor Training Checklists (see Appendices 8.4–8.6 for copies of checklists pertaining to each training component). These checklists break training sessions down into very specific steps and are completed by the supervisor while he or she observes the trainee conduct a practice training session. Then the supervisor and the trainee discuss the steps not completed correctly, and, if necessary, the supervisor models these steps again for the trainee. The trainee then practices these steps until she or he is ready to demonstrate the entire training session.

As with the quizzes, the trainee must perform to criterion before learning a new skill. We consider the criterion met when the trainee can perform the skill two times consecutively without a model, prompt, or correction. Whenever the trainee fails this criterion, the supervisor again models the skill and asks the trainee to imitate it.

Most often, we use simulation for these skill-modeling sessions, but there are two other ways in which this training can proceed. One is direct training. In some instances, it may be appropriate for the trainee to observe an actual training session with a family. The counselor should first ask the parents if they would agree to have an observer present during the training session. For example, during the session before training is to begin, the counselor would explain to the parent that new staff are trained by observing other staff members conducting training. If the parents agree, the trainee would observe an experienced staff member conducting the session. After this, the trainee would then practice conducting a session in a simulated situation while the supervisor observes.

The other way modeling can be done is by showing videotapes of already trained staff performing the skills. The video shows the skills to be performed, and the trainee is asked to demonstrate the skills. The criterion for the trainee to move on to the next skill remains the same, that is, demonstrating the skill two consecutive times without the video. If the trainee fails the criterion, the tape is shown again until the trainee meets the performance criterion.

We have used this way of teaching affective skills to our staff very successfully (McGimsey, Lutzker, & Greene, 1994).

In this training format modeling of the skill is live or by tape. *Role playing* involves the entire sequence of providing the model, having the trainee imitate the model, and having the supervisor provide feedback on the acceptability of the role play (imitation). Feedback involves telling the trainee what skills are being performed correctly and then describing what skills still need to be improved. With the skills that need to be improved, the trainer again models the skills and again asks the trainee to demonstrate that skill. Feedback should always be delivered in a positive manner. The *correct* skill should always be the one that is modeled. The incorrect skill should be pointed out but never modeled. The rationale here is simple: The goal is to learn by seeing the correct behaviors; we do not want to overplay or replay the incorrect skill. It has been said, by way of sports analogy, that a baseball player who is in a hitting slump should view tapes of his performance during the best hitting he has shown rather than focusing on tapes of his batting during the slump. The same goes for the modeling of the skills described here.

Criterion performance refers to ensuring that the performer/trainee can demonstrate the new skill without a model a predetermined number of times before the next skill is taught. For example, before conducting health training, the trainee would be required to demonstrate two complete health training sessions with 95% of the steps completed correctly for at least two consecutive sessions. After this mastery criterion has been achieved, training in home safety skills would then begin.

After the trainee has met criteria for all of the skills in simulation, the next step is to *fade in* actual interactions with the families. Thus the trainee then "shadows" a trained staff member in the homes of the families who are receiving these services. Under the scrutiny of the trained staff member, the trainee is allowed to conduct 10% of the actual delivery of the service to the family. If the trainee meets criterion performance on this, then another 10% is added, until the trainee is delivering the entire session under the supervision of the trained staff member. Once the supervisor and the trainee are comfortable that the trainee demonstrates the skills adequately during a session, the trainee can then handle the sessions without the supervisor.

This fading-in procedure is handled in the same manner as the training previously described. That is, should the trainee falter in home sessions, the supervisor points out what the trainee did correctly and incorrectly, models the skills again, and asks the trainee to show the skills again until the performance criterion is met. The goal of training is always that the trainee masters to the performance criterion whatever skill is being taught.

Fidelity is the process of ensuring that previously mastered skills are maintained over time. Thus periodic fidelity checks on staff performance in the field are an important aspect of staff training from our perspective. During fidelity checks, a supervisor accompanies the staff member to the family's home and observes the staff member. The supervisor uses the same checklist that is used in staff training to record the requisite skills performed by the staff member. After the fidelity session, at the office or in the car, the supervisor reviews the skills that have been maintained to criterion and praises the staff member for the maintenance of those skills. These checklists should be placed in the staff member's file and should be used during quarterly performance reviews.

If any skills have slipped below criterion during the fidelity check, the supervisor reviews them with the staff member. The staff member can be asked at this point if simply discussing the deficits will serve as a reminder and whether the staff member can correct the deficit without further role playing or whether the staff member would like to engage in some role playing with the supervisor in order to refresh the skill. Also, video can be used at this point as an alternative or adjunct to role playing. That is, a video showing some staff member or the staff member under review demonstrating criterion performance in the home can be used to refresh the staff member on the skills that fell below criterion during the fidelity check.

In the case of fidelity "slippage," another fidelity check should be scheduled soon. Family members should be apprised in advance of fidelity checks. The rationale that can be presented to the family is that a supervisor will be attending the next session because this is a routine procedure that allows supervisors to be in touch with families (a true and good reason) and for quality assurance purposes.

Ethnic sensitivity and responsivity represent an extremely important element of staff training. In an increasingly multiethnic culture, this training becomes a necessity (Kapitanoff, Lutzker, & Bigelow, 2000). Even with training in this area, problems of class can arise. In most service projects, even when staff members may be of the same race or ethnic group as families they serve, there may be educational and income differences that separate the staff from the families. In some ways this may be difficult to overcome; however, as with so many aspects of staff training, part of this problem can be solved by exposing staff to the issues of these differences and practicing dialogues that may ease any conflict. Additionally, it may be possible to train and hire staff who are, in fact, in the same community as the families served.

As with other aspects of staff training, ethnic sensitivity can be incorporated into training. Videotapes of experts describing important issues of the ethnic communities served can be used. These tapes can be accompanied by written quizzes covering basic questions from the tapes. For example, a tape on serving the Hispanic community might mention that a counselor should ask a parent's permission before picking up and holding the parent's child. Thus, on the quiz, there would be a question dealing with this issue.

Role playing can also be used in ethnic sensitivity and responsivity training. As with the other role-playing components of staff training, simulated interactions can be held in which the supervisor first demonstrates how to interact and then the staff member/trainee imitates that model. Then the staff member/trainee would be asked to demonstrate five consecutive skills without the need for correction before the performance criterion is considered to be met. Thus, considering the foregoing example, in a simulation, the supervisor would introduce the trainee to Ms. Hernandez and her 3-year-old. Then, among the other skills being reviewed, the supervisor would expect the trainee to compliment Ms. Hernandez on how cute the child is and then ask permission to pick her up.

In many urban areas it may be difficult to find staff and provide training for all of the many cultures represented in that community. For example, more than 50 ethnic groups are more highly concentrated in the Los Angeles area than they are anywhere except in their original countries. Thus, in such cases the issue of ethnic sensitivity remains, and the staff members need to be urged to ask the family to help them learn more about the cultural nuances that may affect the relationship between the staff member and the family and that could help in assisting the staff to provide the best possible service.

Handling common questions from families is another area in which staff can be trained, and such training can go a long way in preventing problematic interactions (Lutzker, 1994). Supervisors can make lists of frequently asked questions and then teach the staff to answer them using their best counseling skills. Also, some of these questions and their respective answers can be addressed in printed materials that can be given to families at the beginning of services and can be reviewed between the family and the staff member.

One of the questions most frequently asked of our staff over the years has been, "Do you have your own children?" Thus, to the parent, the staff member's expertise in dealing with parent–child problems and interactions can be questioned if the service provider does not have her or his own children. We have taught staff, through role playing, to respond to this question by using counseling skills. They are taught to say,

> "I hear a concern on your part about how I can be doing this since I do not have my own children [if, of course, that is the case]. That is an understandable concern. Let me tell you about my training and my supervision. By the way, my supervisor does have children [if that is the case]."

The staff member then goes on to describe supervision and training. Then he or she is encouraged to tell the family member to contact the supervisor if there is ever any question about the expertise and advice of the staff member.

Other questions commonly asked of the counselors have included inquiries about confidentiality and requests for results of questionnaires and observations. Regarding confidentiality, parents are told that everything discussed between the counselor and the family is confidential but that counselors are required by law to report suspicions of possible abuse or neglect. The regulations regarding this mandate are discussed further, and parents are told that they may bring up any questions they have about this at any time in the future. Parents have also indicated that they would like to know the results of assessment observations. Although this information will not be withheld from families, parents are told that after the observation period for any given component is over, all of their questions about how they fared in these assessments will be addressed during the training session.

Staff meetings have several important purposes. It is important for staff to be together to get a sense of the organization and to see the common purposes of the organization. Additionally, much professional development can occur during staff meetings. We recommend the following format for staff meetings:

1. Pass out agenda and minutes
2. Roll call
3. Announcements
4. Feedback
5. Formal case reviews
6. Informal problem solving

7. Special events
8. Business

Agenda items should be sought from the management team during the week prior to the staff meeting. We recommend that staff meetings occur at least weekly. Announcements can, of course, take many forms, such as reminding staff of upcoming events and of whose birthday has occurred during the week. Roll call is important for staff evaluations. If a staff member is frequently tardy or misses staff meetings, this information should be discussed during performance reviews.

We use feedback at staff meetings as a mechanism for ensuring that suggestions made during the previous staff meeting have been given attention. Thus staff and supervisors have feedback forms during meetings . When someone makes a suggestion about what to do with a particular family—for example, a suggestion as to how to help parents improve remembering to state the rules of an activity—that suggestion is written on the feedback form by the staff member whose family is being discussed and by the supervisor who is running the meeting. During the feedback session of the staff meeting the following week, the supervisor asks the staff member whether she or he tried the suggestion and what the outcome was. We have found this strategy effective in increasing the likelihood that staff follows suggestions during meetings, and staff has found that many of the suggestions are then helpful in changing family behavior.

After the follow-through on feedback from the previous meeting, formal case reviews are conducted. Table 8.1 shows the form we use to present cases. A staff member presents a case using this form on a transparency with an overhead projector. The staff member reviews the case and presents the most recent data in graphic or tabular form, also using transparencies. The staff and supervisors then make commentary, ask questions, and make suggestions about the case. Video is also often used to review parent–child interactions. These case presentations ensure that all staff, especially all supervisors, are at least casually familiar with all cases.

Case presentations at staff meetings help improve the quality of services delivered to the family, and at the same time they allow for professional development for the staff member. If a staff member has weak presentational skills, the supervisor can spend time with that person in working on skill improvement in the same manner in which other skills are taught to staff and clients. For example, if a staff member reads notes and does not speak extemporaneously about the case, she or he would receive feedback about this. The supervisor would then model the requisite skill and ask the staff member to imitate it. Before the next presentation, the supervisor would prompt the staff member about the new skills and ask if she or he wants a "rehearsal" before to the next meeting.

After formal case presentations, we recommend an informal problem-solving session in which all staff are encouraged to discuss any clinical or practical issues of concern. These may range from anything such as frustration about parental adherence to a protocol to transportation issues. This "group process" is again useful in team building and problem solving.

We also feel strongly that staff should look forward to staff meetings for a number of reasons. Thus we arrange special events, for example, one or two "big name" speakers each year. In addition to having the speakers make formal presentations, we ask them to participate in a staff meeting. Thus we conduct a staff meeting in its usual manner, and the consultant partici-

TABLE 8.1. Project SafeCare Case Presentation Outline

- Introduce the family (use pseudonyms)
  - Family members (adults and children in the home)
  - Their relationship to each other (parent, stepparent, etc.)
  - Ages
  - Any relevant and specific information regarding background, diagnoses, prior history of drug abuse, maltreatment, etc.
  - Employment
  - Level of education

- Reason for referral: Who referred the family and for what reason.

- Data from indirect measures: Give a brief synopsis of scores and an interpretation of these scores *based on information provided in the appropriate administration/interpretation manual.* If there are discrepancies between your observations and scores on indirect measures, address them.
  - Child Abuse Potential Inventory
  - Beck Depression Inventory
  - Parenting Stress Index
  - Eyberg Child Behavior Inventory
  - Parent Behavior Checklist
  - Parental Anger Inventory
  - Conners' Rating Scales

- Data from direct measures: Present the graphed data (use transparencies so all can see the data) and an interpretation of the data. Include data from all three training components.

- Provide a brief description of any relevant information related to assessment or training and of progress made to date.

pates in the same feedback and problem solving as the rest of the staff. We have found this strategy very popular with staff, who remark that they feel quite validated by having the attention of prestigious consultants.

The final component of staff meetings is routine business. This is the point in a meeting at which the practical aspects of service delivery get discussed, schedules are planned, and paperwork is turned in. Because staff occasionally miss meetings, minutes from the meetings, including the business items need to be distributed.

Professional development is another important aspect of staff training and development. Bringing in outside experts for consultation often serves two purposes for staff. First, it provides a fresh perspective and new information. It can also serve to validate for staff that they are, in fact, doing good, effective work. Supporting and encouraging staff attendance at local, regional, and national conferences is also an important aspect of staff development and training. Attendance at these events serves similar purposes to bringing in consultants, in that at these events staff are at once exposed to state-of-the-art research and service in child maltreatment prevention or treatment and also often reassured in learning that their own work is valuable.

Staff training and development are key to successful services. A well-trained, supported, well-motivated staff keeps a project viable. The belief that staff training should always be a developmental and dynamic process goes a long way in achieving the goal of being well trained and motivated.

HANDLING SETBACKS

Inevitably there are setbacks with any given family. These may include poor performance, canceled appointments, or outright refusal to participate in one of the intervention protocols. Actually, once a family has committed to these intervention services, we find surprisingly few setbacks. We believe this is due to the succinct nature of the interventions and the fact that we focus on teaching skills rather than on "talk therapy." Nonetheless, attrition that occurs before services are rendered has been a serious problem for us and for other professionals providing in-home interventions in child maltreatment. To overcome this problem, several changes probably need to be made before any interventions are offered and presented. One change that we have posited and believe might make a difference is to use former participants in the project as trainers. That is, we would teach parents who successfully participated in receiving the intervention to be teachers themselves of the intervention protocols. We believe that these parents would help bridge cultural and educational barriers that may be one of the reasons for attrition.

The advantage of these highly structured protocols is to provide few reasons why parents could not learn to be effective teachers themselves. To do this would require not only that they master the protocols but also that they master the teaching skills. We would then strongly suggest that fidelity of the parents' teaching skills and subsequent efficacy with other parents be closely monitored.

Help can and should also be solicited from the child protective service agencies in pushing families toward cooperating with these kinds of intervention programs. Agency personnel should explain to families that cooperating with these skills training programs means potentially less scrutiny from the service agencies.

The most effective mechanism we have found with families who may be faltering in one or more components of a protocol is to have them practice only the part of the skill with which they are having difficulty. Actually, another "interesting" strategy that we have also found occasionally effective is to remind the family that the faster they master the skills, the sooner we are able to extricate ourselves from their lives.

Of course, there may be situations in families' lives that make it difficult for them to follow through with training. For this reason, it is important for counselors to be able to engage in problem solving with the family to help determine if there are other steps that must be taken before training can be resumed. For example, if a parent is having difficulties paying bills and rent and is worried about the possibility that the family will be evicted, this matter is clearly of a high priority. Having the ability to provide referrals to other agencies that may be able to help or simply talking through some potential solutions may not only allow the parent to focus again on training but also provide a valuable service to families. Additionally, this may reassure the family that the counselor is truly concerned with their well-being and willing to offer assistance in any possible manner.

COUNSELOR QUALITIES

Offering suggestions about the qualities of good counselors can be risky for several reasons, but the primary reason is that we have found that personality characteristics and individual style can vary greatly among effective counselors. For example, we have found that both exuberance and a quiet style can each be effective. Whether a counselor's personality falls at either extreme or in the middle, however, we have found that the ability to express a certain degree of enthusiasm to families is an essential quality of a counselor.

An ability to handle some of the frustrations of working with families who are often less than adherent and who present many challenges is another essential characteristic, although it is a difficult one to gauge in an applicant for such a position. Wanting to "do good" but understanding that good is done in the form of skills training rather than through talk therapy is another good quality of a counselor. Yet the counselor must clearly demonstrate good empathy and ability to reflect that empathy to families. These skills can be measured, just as many of the other skills discussed here can be.

The ability to work independently is a valuable characteristic. Once trained, counselors' contact with coworkers and supervisors may be infrequent, as most of the counselor's time is spent with families in their homes. The ability to manage a caseload of families, to schedule and keep regular meetings, and to keep up-to-date on data collection and other record-keeping duties is very important.

Finally, the ability to handle stressful or challenging situations can be a most valuable quality of a counselor. Often, families reported for child maltreatment experience multiple stressors. This situation can result in significant challenges for a counselor attempting to meet with the family on a weekly basis. Families have been known not to show up for scheduled meetings, to move without leaving contact information, and to be highly resistant to assistance. Persistence in following up with families is important here, but it is equally important not to take such behavior personally, as long as the counselor has made every effort to gain rapport and build a relationship with the family. It is also crucial for supervisors to build a supportive working environment in which frustrations, as well as achievements, can be discussed openly and in which everyone can learn from others' experiences. Providing an enriching environment for counselors can ultimately benefit families by helping to retain quality staff, to reduce staff turnover, and to develop counselors' skills.

SUMMARY AND CONCLUSIONS

In this book we present a set of protocols and rationales for offering in-home direct skills training that has been effective in teaching these skills to families involved in or at high risk for child maltreatment. In no way do we suggest that this is a panacea, but we have found that new skills are learned and that risks of future or first-time child maltreatment have been dramatically reduced. We believe that it is important to try to remain true to the protocols as they have been presented. We have no data or experience as to the efficacy of these protocols if adjustments are made to them.

The literature on intervention and prevention in child maltreatment clearly shows that these families frequently need help with parenting skills, child health care skills, and home safety and cleanliness. Our own research has shown that offering these protocols clearly teaches the skills to families who participate fully; as a result there is usually a reduction in parental depression and stress and measurable reductions in risk to the children of these families.

Needless to say, the skills suggested here are not the only skills that provide help for parents and children involved in child maltreatment. Stress reduction skills may be very useful, and a number of protocols are available in the literature for providing such training. We would emphasize, however, that if you search for such programs, you should ensure that the stress reduction protocols are empirically validated.

Although the material presented in this book focuses on the parent, the child often needs intervention because of having been the victim of maltreatment. Again, we would recommend the professional literature in looking for effective, *empirically validated* procedures.

Many have asked us if it is frustrating to work in child maltreatment. Surely, there can be many frustrations with the families, with the system, and with the circumstances that promote child maltreatment, but we have actually been buoyed by seeing the successful behavior change in the majority of the families we have seen and in hearing their excitement and pleasure with the changes they have effected. We hope that this book is helpful in allowing others to experience these kinds of rewards.

Parent–Child Interaction Staff Training Quizzes and Answers

After reading all applicable assessment or training materials, you must pass these quizzes at 90% correct in order to move on to the next segment of staff training, which is modeling and practice of the target assessment or training procedures.

Assessment Protocol Quiz

This quiz is for use with the time-sampling method of assessing parent and child interaction skills. This quiz may be modified to be applicable to a different method of assessment, such as a checklist.

A. Please indicate True (T) or False (F).
   1. ___ Within a partial-interval time-sampling procedure, the behavior must occur a minimum of two times before being recorded.
   2. ___ The observer should try to become involved in the parent–child interaction as quickly as possible to prevent the child from being distracted by the presence of a stranger.
   3. ___ When a parent makes a verbal statement to a child, it may need to be scored as several different behaviors.

B. Please fill in the blanks.
   1. If a child refuses to wear a specific article of clothing, and she or he throws it at the mother and flails violently, this is scored as _____.
   2. _____ means that a child begins an appropriately requested behavior within 30 seconds of the first appropriate instruction from the adult.
   3. When a child makes verbalizations in which she is giggling and laughing, she is scored as demonstrating _____ affect.
   4. _____ means that a parent expands on a statement or action made by the child, suggests ways to expand the activity, and gives the child command of direction in an activity.
   5. When the parent tells the child what is expected of him or her throughout the activity before beginning a new activity, this is scored as _____.
   6. _____ means that a parent hits or grabs the child harshly.

C. Please circle the correct response.
   1. If a child repeatedly calls for a parent in a whining or demanding voice ("Mom, mom, mom . . . "), it is scored as:
      a. inappropriate verbal.
      b. aggression.
      c. negative affect.
      d. following instructions.
      e. a and c.
      f. b and c.
   2. If a child says to his mother, "You're so stupid!" while giggling and smiling at her, it is scored as:
      a. appropriate verbal, positive affect.
      b. appropriate verbal, negative affect.

(continued)

    c. inappropriate verbal, positive affect.

    d. inappropriate verbal, negative affect.

3. If a parent hugs the child while he or she is sitting on the parent's lap, this is scored as:

    a. incidental teaching.

    b. appropriate touch.

    c. appropriate proximity.

    d. leveling.

    e. a and c.

    f. b and d.

4. If a parent expands on a statement made by the child or provides additional information related to the activity or topic of conversation in which the child is engaged, such as, "Then the bees make honey from the nectar," this is scored as:

    a. explanation and prompting.

    b. explaining activity and appropriate verbal.

    c. appropriate verbal and incidental teaching.

    d. feedback and explaining activity.

    e. appropriate verbal and feedback.

    f. feedback only.

5. "Sue, now it is time to clean up. You need to pick up all of these blocks, and then we can go outside." (Waits for response).

    This is scored as:

    a. appropriate verbal.

    b. explain activity.

    c. explain rules.

    d. explain consequences.

    e. appropriate instruction.

    f. all of the above.

D. Match the behavior to the example. There may be more than one correct response per question.

1. ___Parent: (Screaming) "Stop doing that this minute, or else!"

2. ___Child: Screaming, striking, grabbing, kicking, biting.

3. ___Parent: Kneels down to make eye contact with the child.

4. ___Parent: "If you come into the house, we can read a book."

5. ___Child: (Laughing) "Mom, stop tickling me!"

6. ___Parent: (After child points out a dog) "What color is the dog?"

7. ___Child: Performs appropriate behavior within 30 seconds of appropriate instructions from parent.

8. ___Parent: "You put your toys away very neatly."

9. ___Parent: (While drawing with the child) "You're drawing big circles."

    a. inappropriate verbal

    b. positive affect

    c. leveling

    d. appropriate verbal

    e. following instructions

    f. inappropriate instructions

    g. explain consequences

    h. incidental teaching

(continued)

    i. negative affect
    j. provide appropriate performance feedback
    k. physical aggression

Answers to Assessment Protocol Quiz

A. True or False (1 point each)
    1. F
    2. F
    3. T

B. Fill in the blanks (1 point each)
    1. aggression
    2. following instructions
    3. positive
    4. incidental teaching
    5. explaining the rules
    6. inappropriate touch

C. Multiple choice (1 point each)
    1. e
    2. c
    3. f
    4. c
    5. f

D. Match the columns (1 point for each item; total of 17)
    1. a, f
    2. a, i, k
    3. c
    4. d, g
    5. b, d
    6. d, h
    7. e
    8. d, j
    9. d, h

Parent–Child Interactions Training Protocol Quiz
This quiz is to be used in combination with the Planned Activities Training Quiz.

A. Fill in the blanks
    1. The methods described in the general training protocol that are to be used in each training session include _____, _____, _____, and _____.
    2. Before beginning training, the counselor should provide a _____ for the training.
    3. Activity cards are given to parents to _____.
    4. When providing feedback to parents about their performance, the counselor should always provide _____ feedback first, and then deliver _____ feedback.

(continued)

B. Please indicate True (T) or False (F).
1. ___ The basic rationale for PAT is that, because it is not possible to prevent some challenging behaviors, it is important to have a plan for dealing with difficult behavior.
2. ___ Training should be conducted only in the family's home.
3. ___ The first session should involve a discussion of all of the steps of PAT.

Answers to PCI Training Protocol Quiz

A. Fill in the Blanks
1. instructions or explanation of target behavior with a rationale; modeling; parent practice; and feedback with additional practice (4 points).
2. rationale (1 point).
3. prompt them to engage their child in daily living and play activities using PAT and good interaction skills so that positive parent–child interactions are promoted (1 point).
4. positive; corrective (2 points).

B. Please indicate True (T) or False (F) (1 point each).
1. False
2. False
3. True

Planned Activities Training Quiz
1. What is the rationale for Planned Activities Training (PAT)?
2. Name 8 of the 10 basic components (or steps) of PAT.
3. There are many settings in which PAT can be assessed and trained. Name one community and three home settings.
4. Describe how PAT would be used in one of these settings, using each step of PAT.

Answers to Planned Activities Training Quiz
1. Prevention is better than a cure. When parents keep children engaged in activities and make the rules clear, children are more likely to maintain good behavior, and inappropriate behavior is prevented (1 point).
2. Identify difficult settings or situations; prepare in advance; explain activities; explain rules; explain consequences; provide engaging activities; incidental teaching; give choices; provide feedback, provide consequences; use positive interaction skills (8 points; any of these or close approximations of these are accepted).
3. Home settings: mealtime, bath time, bedtime, playtime, getting ready to go out, having guests over, clean-up time, and so forth.
   Community settings: grocery store; friends' or relatives' homes; doctor's and dentist's office; shopping; in the car; waiting rooms; restaurants, and so forth (4 points).
4. Any example which incorporates all of the components of the parent–child interactions skills protocol, including good interaction skills and PAT, will be accepted. Score according to the number of steps represented out of a possible total of 10 points.

Home Safety and Cleanliness Counselor Training Quizzes and Answers

After reading all applicable assessment or training materials, you must pass these quizzes at 90% correct in order to move on to the next segment of staff training, which is modeling and practice of the target assessment or training procedures.

HAPI-R Assessment Protocol Quiz
 1. List the four possible conditions that make an object accessible.
 2. If a box contains 34 books of matches, how would you score this object?
 3. What is the distance between the wall and an electrical plate that would indicate the item should be scored as a hazard?
 4. If the top of a kitchen counter measures 35 inches from the floor, how tall does a child have to be, from feet to eye level, to be able to climb onto the counter?
 5. State the scoring rule when you observe a six-pack of beer.
 6. How is roll of Saran Wrap that is not in its original box scored?
 7. How is an accessible tablecloth stored in a plastic bag scored?
 8. How is a can of paint found in a child's bedroom scored if the lid is securely fitted and will not come off unless pried with an opener?
 9. How is a stereo speaker wire scored?
10. How is a crib scored when it is within 2 feet of a cord and is filled with objects and used as a storage area?
11. How is an electrical plate scored when it is taped to the wall and cannot move?
12. Under what category of hazards is jewelry cleaner scored?
13. Under what category of hazards is mouthwash scored?
14. Under what category of hazards is antiperspirant scored?
15. How is a television set cord scored when the set is unplugged and stored on a closet shelf?
16. How are steel wool pads scored when they contain no soap?
17. Under what category of hazards is a box of Mr. Bubble bubble bath scored?
18. Under what category of hazards is a bottle of liquid Woolite scored?
19. How do you determine whether a child can climb onto a surface or shelf?
20. How would you measure the accessibility of a kitchen counter with drawers and cabinets below the counter?
21. Describe how shelves or other objects can be stair-steps, and give an example found in the bathroom.
22. How is a "step-up" defined when trying to determine accessibility?
23. Under which category is a broken window scored?
24. A 3-year-old has a reach of 42 inches. There are several small objects on the dresser in his parents' room. The height of the dresser is 42 inches. Are the objects scored as hazards? Why or why not?
25. Name the eight categories of hazards and give an example of each.

Answers to HAPI-R Assessment Protocol Quiz (1 point each)
 1. A child can reach it while standing on the floor.
    A child can reach it while standing on an adjacent object.
    The object is in an unlocked space.
    An object does not have a childproof lock or the cap or lock is broken.

(continued)

2. 1 fire hazard
3. 1/4 inch
4. 35 inches
5. 1 alcoholic beverage
6. 1 plastic
7. It is not scored.
8. 1 paints and stains
9. Stereo speaker wire is not scored as an electrical hazard because it carries a very low current that cannot result in shock. As a crib cord, it is counted only if it is suspended above an area where the child might play. If the wire is flat on the floor, it is not counted.
10. It is not scored because it is not in a designated sleep or play area.
11. It is not scored.
12. Detergents and cleansers
13. Liquid medication
14. Beauty products
15. It is not scored because it is unplugged and not operational.
16. If small enough to fit in a choke tube or empty toilet roll, it would be a small ingestible object.
17. Beauty products
18. Detergents and cleansers
19. A child can climb onto any surface that is below a child's eye level. A child can step up or climb onto a series of progressively higher surfaces if they are arranged in a stair-step fashion and are lower than the child's eye level when the child is standing on each preceding surface level.
20. If the child can open cupboards or drawers and use them to climb up in a stair-step fashion to higher surfaces, measure from the highest surface onto which the child can climb.
21. The child can step on the medicine cabinet shelf under the sink or climb onto the toilet in order to reach up onto the bathroom counter or climb to higher surfaces.
22. A step-up is a surface onto which the child can climb to reach higher surfaces. Do not score surfaces as accessible under the assumption that a child could move an object allowing him or her a step up to that surface.
23. Broken glass would be scored as a sharp object. If the child can reach and can fit through the window, it is a falling hazard in the "windows" category.
24. Yes. The height of the dresser is 42", and the child's reach is 42". If the child can reach any portion of the top surface of the dresser, then all items on top of the dresser are accessible.
25. Fire and electrical hazards
    Hazardous ingestible small objects
    Hazardous mechanical objects
    Firearm hazards
    Solid and liquid poisonous hazards
    Hazardous sharp object hazards
    Falling hazards
    Drowning hazards
    (Check examples against definitions in manual.)

CLEAN Assessment Protocol Quiz
1. What is the CLEAN?
2. Define the scoring criteria for the following.
    Clean
    Clothes/linens
    Items not belonging

(continued)

  3. What does "ODM" stand for? List three examples.
  4. Cite the "room specific rules" for the following.
     Dirty dishes
     Mealtime dishes
     Toys
     Splashed water
     Dirty sheets without stains
  5. What information is required at the top of each CLEAN data sheet?
  6. What is an "item area"? List three examples.
  7. How many checks should be made per item area on the data sheet?
  8. Give an example of an appropriate "comment" for the kitchen.
  9. How are roaches quantified using the CLEAN?
 10. List the three dimensions of the CLEAN using the numeric weights assigned to each.
 11. State the "decision rule" for each of the following:
     A pile of papers
     Spiderwebs
     Dog feces
 12. Before beginning a home cleanliness assessment, what should be obtained?
 13. What are some examples of basic cleaning supplies?
 14. What is a CLEAN composite score?
 15. If a room scores a 95% composite score, what does this mean?

Answers to CLEAN Assessment Protocol Quiz (1 point each)
  1. Checklist of Living Environments to Assess Neglect
  2. Clean: Less than 1 square inch of ODM or NOM in direct contact with each item area
     Clothes/linens: Any article worn by a person or any cloth or material other than clothes
     Items not belonging: Any object that can be thrown away or has a more appropriate storage space.
  3. Organic decaying matter: spilled food, grease spots, crumbs
  4. Dirty dishes: piled over counter level, count as items not belonging
     Mealtime dishes: Not counted if observation occurs during mealtime
     Toys: Two toys per child are acceptable, or if child has a set up and consolidated play area that is used regularly. Otherwise, count as items not belonging.
     Splashed water: Scored as clean, unless water contains ODM
     Dirty sheets without stains: Scored as dirty. If located somewhere other than on bed, counted as clothes/linens not belonging.
  5. Family; observer; date; room; session; phase (baseline, treatment, or follow-up); and general condition of room (+, −, O)
  6. An item area is an area that has discrete and observable boundaries, such as chairs, bookcases, tables, couches, sinks, refrigerators, area rugs, furniture items, and so forth.
  7. Three
  8. "In general, your kitchen looks very good. The only problem I noticed was that your garbage is without a cover and there are crumbs on the counter. Everything else looks just fine."
  9. The CLEAN does not quantify live bugs. If they are dead, score as ODM.
 10. Clean (10); Dirty (0)
     Clothes/linens: 0 = 5 points; 1–5 = 4 points; 6–10 = 3 points; 11–15 = 2 points; 16–20 = 1 point; 20 or more = 0 points.
     Objects not belonging: 0 = 5 points; 1–5 = 4 points; 6–10 = 3 points; 11–15 = 2 points; 16–20 = 1 point; 20 or more = 0 points.

(continued)

11. One object not belonging
    Dirty/NOM
    Dirty/ODM
12. The informed consent form, which informs parents of their rights and indicates agreement on which areas the counselor may observe
13. Broom, mop, dustpan, vacuum, dust rag, paper towels, toilet brush, glass and surface cleaner, laundry detergent, and so forth.
14. This score summarizes the whole room's condition.
15. The room is generally very clean. 100% is the highest score possible.

Safety and Cleanliness Training Protocol Quiz
 1. What should occur in the home before the start of training?
 2. What materials do you need to bring to training?
 3. List the dimensions of cleanliness that are reviewed at each training session.
 4. Describe how you determine the height and reach of the child.
 5. Describe the three methods for making hazards inaccessible that are reviewed at every session.
 6. Describe the four components that should be part of any training session.
 7. Describe the rationale for home safety and cleanliness training.
 8. Describe two different strategies for prompting parents to complete "homework" assignments.
 9. How does Session 5 differ from the other sessions?
10. How is the room in which training is conducted on any given session determined?

Answers to Safety and Cleanliness Training Protocol Quiz (1 point each)
 1. Consent form discussed with parent and signed and baseline observations
 2. Data sheets; pencil; tape measure; choke tube; safety devices (if provided); cleaning supplies (if provided); screwdriver (for installing safety devices)
 3. Clean/dirty; Clothes/linens; Objects not belonging
 4. Measure the child while he or she is standing with feet flat on the floor. Obtain measure of eye level by measuring child from floor to eye level. Obtain measure of reach by measuring child from floor to tip of fingers when arm is reaching straight up above the child's head.
 5. Use of child-resistant closures; locking up items; placing items out of child's reach.
 6. Instructions with rationale, modeling, practice, and feedback with additional practice.
 7. Making your home clean and safe can prevent serious accidents.
 8. Give verbal instructions; leave a written list of instructions; leave a Polaroid picture of areas to be cleaned or hazards to be removed; and so forth.
 9. This is a review session. If training was conducted in four rooms, the fifth session involves a review of the training conducted in these rooms.
10. The room that is the dirtiest and has the most hazards is the first room in which training is conducted.

Health Counselor Training Quizzes and Answers

After reading all applicable assessment or training materials, you must pass these quizzes at 90% correct in order to move on to the next segment of staff training, which is modeling and practice of the target assessment or training procedures.

Health Parent Behavior Checklist Quiz

A. Fill in the blanks
  1. Before conducting baseline observations with the parent, it is important to provide them with a _____ for the observations.
  2. Parents' health care skills are assessed in two ways: by conducting a _____ and a _____.
  3. The materials needed for an observation include:

  _____   _____   _____

  _____   _____   _____

  4. When completing the Parent Behavior Checklist, for each step completed correctly record a ____, and for each step completed incorrectly record a ____.
  5. For each step on the Parent Behavior Checklist that does not apply to the particular scenario, ____ should be recorded in the appropriate space.
  6. When calling the physician, which five steps should the parent follow?

  _____   _____   _____

  _____   _____   _____

  7. Before administering medication to a child, the parent must _____.
  8. When administering medication to the child, if the instructions on the label and in the reference book conflict, the parent should follow the instructions from the _____.
  9. If a parent skips a step on the Parent Behavior Checklist but then demonstrates the next step correctly, a _____ is scored for the skipped step and a _____ is scored for the next step.

B. True or false
  1. ___ When treating a child at home, the parent should stop treatment when the symptoms are gone instead of continuing treatment for however long the reference book or doctor suggests.
  2. ___ As long as the parent is following the directions in the reference book exactly, he or she does not have to record the symptoms and treatment on the recording chart.
  3. ___ It is important for the parent to have the child nearby when calling the doctor, in case he or she wants the parent to look for additional symptoms.
  4. ___ The role-play scenarios contain true–false questions.
  5. ___ If a parent says she would call the doctor in a particular situation, the counselor should role play this phone call with her to make sure that she knows the steps to follow and can provide the doctor with important information.
  6. ___ It is not important for a parent to demonstrate how he would do the steps he describes for his child's health care as long as he knows the proper order of the steps to follow.

(continued)

7. ___ Before telling you how she would deal with her child's health problem, the parent should explain the problem presented on the scenario card as she understood it.

8. ___ When a parent appears to be finished with the role play, the counselor should ask if there is anything else he would do. If he says there is nothing else he would do, he should be prompted to take the next step in the reference book.

9. ___ An appropriate response when seeking emergency treatment would be to call 911 for help.

10. ___ If a parent records the treatment that she administers to her child in a place other than the health manual or recording chart, score it as correct.

Answers to Parent Behavior Checklist Quiz

A. Fill in the blanks
   1. rationale (1 point)
   2. True–false quiz; role-play scenario (2 points)
   3. Parent Behavior Checklist-Counselor's Version; true–false quiz; role-play scenario cards; role-play scenario answer sheet; doll or child; related medical supplies (if provided to parents) (5 points)
   4. +, – (2 points)
   5. N/A (1 point)
   6. recording chart ready; have pencil; child nearby; describe symptoms; follow physician's instructions (5 points)
   7. read instructions on label or in reference book (1 point)
   8. label (1 point)
   9. –, + (2 points)

B. True or False (1 point each)
   1. False
   2. False
   3. True
   4. False
   5. True
   6. False
   7. True
   8. False
   9. True
   10. True

Health Training Protocol Quiz

A. Fill in the blanks
   1. The health manual includes sections such as: _____; _____; and _____.
   2. In addition to teaching parents to identify and treat their children's illnesses, the health manual and health training also teach parents tips for _____.
   3. Parents should be provided with two types of feedback on their performance during training. These are _____ and _____.
   4. In addition to explaining and modeling steps for parents, the counselor should give parents ample opportunities for _____.

(continued)

B. Indicate true or false
  1. ___ At the end of each health training session, a homework assignment is given to parents, and they are asked to memorize the steps in the next chapter of the health manual.
  2. ___ A rationale for the training must be provided for parents at the beginning of every health training session.
  3. ___ To ensure that parents are familiar with all of the steps in the Parent Behavior Checklist and are capable of carrying them out properly, parents are asked to continue practicing steps that they have already performed adequately.
  4. ___ Parents should not be given too much positive feedback so that they do not become overconfident in their abilities and stop following the instructions in the health manual.
  5. ___ As part of the training, the counselor helps the parents prepare a plan of action in case their child becomes sick at a later date.
  6. ___ If a counselor is confident that parents are reading the manual as assigned, it is not necessary to review the content with them.

Answers to health Training Protocol Quiz

A. Fill in the blanks
  1. Possible responses include: recording chart for parents, lists of illnesses and treatments, steps for treating illnesses at home, calling the doctor, and emergency situations, or any of the chapter headings, such as "Planning and Prevention." (3 points)
  2. keeping their children healthy (1 point)
  3. positive; corrective (2 points)
  4. practice

B. True or False (1 point each)
  1. False
  2. True
  3. False
  4. False
  5. True
  6. False

Parent–Child Interaction Training Sessions 1–4 Counselor Training Checklist

Staff member _____   Date _____   Observ. # _____

+ correct
– incorrect

Staff member has materials ready			
Activity cards	+	–	N/A
Fun time board (or other type of card organizer)	+	–	N/A
Toys (as needed)	+	–	N/A
PAT checklist (1–play; 2–3–daily living activities)	+	–	N/A
PCI data sheet	+	–	N/A
Tape player & headphones/10-second-obs, 5-sec-rec tape	+	–	N/A
Observer conducts one PCI/PAT observation	+	–	N/A
Counselor provides rationale for training (specific to target activity)			
Increase positive interactions	+	–	N/A
Provide parents with skills to plan age approp. & stimulating activities	+	–	N/A
Increase bonding and attachment	+	–	N/A
Teach appropriate behavior, play skills, and communication to child	+	–	N/A
Prevent challenging child behavior	+	–	N/A
* Counselor provides feedback on pretraining observation			
* Provide positive, descriptive praise	+	–	N/A
* Provide instructions regarding skills needing improvement	+	–	N/A
* Model skills that could be improved on	+	–	N/A
* Parent practices these skills again	+	–	N/A
* Provide positive, descriptive praise	+	–	N/A
* Provide further instructions	+	–	N/A
Counselor makes sure parent has materials			
Relevant activity cards	+	–	N/A
Toys (as needed)	+	–	N/A
Supplies relevant to the activity (towels, clothes)	+	–	N/A
Appropriate PAT checklist	+	–	N/A

* Not applicable during first session

(continued)

Counselor provides overview of session			
Tell parent you will discuss and model each step during the activity	+	–	N/A
Tell parent she or he will then have opportunity to practice	+	–	N/A
Counselor provides a description/rationale for each target behavior			
Provide descrip. of interaction skills (see obs. data for skills that are lacking)	+	–	N/A
Provide rationale for each interaction skill discussed	+	–	N/A
Answer parent's questions	+	–	N/A
Encourage parents' ideas and suggestions (what do they already do well?)	+	–	N/A
Counselor describes each step of the PAT checklist	+	–	N/A
Provide rationale for each PAT step	+	–	N/A
Answer parent's questions	+	–	N/A
Encourage parents' ideas and suggestions (what do they already do well?)	+	–	N/A
Counselor models interaction skills and PAT			
Model interaction skills/PAT during an activity (point out specific skills)	+	–	N/A
Point out specific skills as they are demonstrated	+	–	N/A
Demonstrate only a few behaviors at a time (depends on parent's skill level)	+	–	N/A
Parent practices interaction skills and PAT			
Ask parent to practice the skills just observed (in same activity or new one)	+	–	N/A
Provide prompts as needed	+	–	N/A
Counselor provides positive and corrective feedback to parent			
Provide positive, descriptive praise	+	–	N/A
Provide instructions regarding skills needing improvement	+	–	N/A
Model skills that could be improved on	+	–	N/A
Parent practices these skills again	+	–	N/A
Provide positive, descriptive praise	+	–	N/A
Provide further instructions	+	–	N/A
Repeat instr., rationale, modeling, practice, & feedback for remaining skills	+	–	N/A
Help parent identify skills to be practiced in coming week (written reminders)	+	–	N/A
Help parent decide on activity cards to be used in the coming week	+	–	N/A
Reviews what was completed this session	+	–	N/A
Provides general, positive feedback about the session	+	–	N/A
Reminds parents to use skills they have just practiced while interacting with child	+	–	N/A
Reminds parents to use activity cards as reminders for fun, engaging activities	+	–	N/A
Total +			
Total + and –			
Percent correct			

Home Safety and Cleanliness Training Sessions 1–4 Counselor Training Checklist

Staff member _____   Date _____   Observ. # _____

+ correct
− incorrect

Staff member has appropriate materials ready			
Data sheets	+	−	N/A
Tape measure (used to demonstrate reach and eye level)	+	−	N/A
Choke tube or empty toilet paper roll (used to determine hazardous small objects)	+	−	N/A
Safety devices	+	−	N/A
Pretraining observation	+	−	N/A
Rationale			
Childproof home	+	−	N/A
Prevent accidents	+	−	N/A
Home is healthier and safer	+	−	N/A
Training takes place over several sessions	+	−	N/A
Involves looking through home	+	−	N/A
Instructions			
Training takes place in one room at a time	+	−	N/A
"Today we will work on reducing hazards and cleaning the _____"	+	−	N/A
* Feedback about scores from previous observations	+	−	N/A
* Positive feedback for desired changes	+	−	N/A
* If unsafe or unclean:			
* Provide corrective feedback	+	−	N/A
* Locate areas not yet clean or safe	+	−	N/A
* Help parent correct items or make plan to do so	+	−	N/A
* Have parent correct items at that time	+	−	N/A
* Give additional feedback as needed	+	−	N/A
Introduce cleanliness training			
Describe three dimensions of cleanliness	+	−	N/A
Ask parent to restate three dimensions	+	−	N/A
Discuss general cleaning methods	+	−	N/A
Locate cleaning supplies (or instruct parent to obtain them if not provided)	+	−	N/A

* Not applicable during first session

(continued)

Introduce safety training			
Review three methods for making hazards inaccessible	+	–	N/A
Demonstrate how to determine child's eye level and reach	+	–	N/A
Review eight categories of hazards	+	–	N/A
Ask parent to restate three methods, measurement, and eight categories	+	–	N/A
Describe use of safety devices	+	–	N/A
Provide feedback about score in current room	+	–	N/A
Identify specific categories present in current room	+	–	N/A
Locate one item or area and demonstrate how to make clean and safe	+	–	N/A
Provide safety devices/cleaning supplies as needed	+	–	N/A
Model making area clean and safe	+	–	N/A
Prompt parent to practice	+	–	N/A
Provide positive and corrective feedback	+	–	N/A
Prompt parent to identify additional unsafe or unclean areas	+	–	N/A
Prompt parent to make area clean and safe	+	–	N/A
Gradually reduce your instructions/prompts based on parent's performance	+	–	N/A
Repeat instructions, modeling, practice, and feedback for all remaining hazards	+	–	N/A
Address all hazards in the room (through training and/or assignment)	+	–	N/A
Provide feedback	+	–	N/A
Give assignment for making additional areas safe and clean	+	–	N/A
Review hazards or unclean areas that remain	+	–	N/A
If necessary, leave additional prompt to complete assignment	+	–	N/A
Ask parent to keep current room and previously trained rooms safe and clean	+	–	N/A
Total +			
Total + and –			
Percent correct			

Health Training Session 1
Counselor Training Checklist

Staff member _____   Date _____   Observ. # _____

+ correct
− incorrect

Staff member has appropriate materials ready			
True–false quiz	+	−	N/A
Health manual	+	−	N/A
Scenario cards and answer sheets	+	−	N/A
Health Recording Chart	+	−	N/A
Parent Behavior Checklist (Counselor's Version)	+	−	N/A
Doll	+	−	N/A
Health supplies	+	−	N/A
Conducts true–false quiz correctly	+	−	N/A
Conducts "treat at home" scenario with no prompts	+	−	N/A
Provides rationale for health training			
Keep your children healthy	+	−	N/A
Recognize and treat illness or injury	+	−	N/A
Learn when and how to call the doctor or seek emergency treatment	+	−	N/A
Use reference materials	+	−	N/A
Keep good health records	+	−	N/A
Makes sure parent has appropriate materials			
Health manual	+	−	N/A
Health Recording Chart	+	−	N/A
Parent Behavior Checklist (Parent's Version)	+	−	N/A
Pen or pencil	+	−	N/A
Provides description of the training session			
Will discuss steps parent can follow to identify and treat illness	+	−	N/A
Will show an example of how to follow each step	+	−	N/A
Then parent will have opportunity to practice steps	+	−	N/A
Conduct discussion of each step of the Parent Beh. Checklist (see definitions)	+	−	N/A
Answers parent's questions	+	−	N/A
Models steps of Parent Beh. Checklist using a novel "treat-at-home" scenario	+	−	N/A
Answers parent's questions	+	−	N/A
Parent practices with same scenario as demonstrated	+	−	N/A

(continued)

Counselor provides positive and corrective feedback to parent			
Provides positive, descriptive praise	+	–	N/A
Provides instructions regarding steps not correct or incomplete	+	–	N/A
Models steps as appropriate	+	–	N/A
Parent practices again steps that were incorrect or incomplete	+	–	N/A
Provides additional feedback as necessary until correct	+	–	N/A
Answers parent's questions	+	–	N/A
Counselor reviews health manual with parent (first chapter only)			
Discuss material	+	–	N/A
Answer parent's questions	+	–	N/A
Complete exercises	+	–	N/A
Demonstrate new skills	+	–	N/A
Parent practices new skills	+	–	N/A
Provides feedback to parent	+	–	N/A
Reviews what was competed during the session	+	–	N/A
Provides general feedback about session	+	–	N/A
Reminds parents to use what they have learned so far when child is ill	+	–	N/A
Asks parent to read next chapter of health manual before next mtg.	+	–	N/A
Total +			
Total + and –			
Percent correct			

Health Training Sessions 2 and 3 Counselor Training Checklist

Staff member _____   Date _____   Observ. # _____

+ correct
− incorrect

Staff member has appropriate materials ready			
True–false quiz	+	−	N/A
Health manual	+	−	N/A
Scenario cards and answer sheets	+	−	N/A
Health Recording Chart	+	−	N/A
Parent Behavior Checklist (Counselor's Version)	+	−	N/A
Doll	+	−	N/A
Health supplies	+	−	N/A
Conducts true–false quiz correctly	+	−	N/A
Conducts "treat at home" scenario with no prompts	+	−	N/A
Makes sure parent has all of the appropriate materials			
Health manual	+	−	N/A
Health Recording Chart	+	−	N/A
Parent Behavior Checklist (Parent's Version)	+	−	N/A
Pen or pencil	+	−	N/A
Provides positive and corrective feedback			
Provides positive, descriptive praise	+	−	N/A
Provides instructions regarding steps not correct or incomplete	+	−	N/A
Models steps as appropriate	+	−	N/A
Parent practices again steps that were incorrect or incomplete	+	−	N/A
Provides additional feedback as necessary until correct	+	−	N/A
Answers parent's questions	+	−	N/A
Provides rationale and description of remainder of session			
Session 2—Plan ahead for when your children are sick	+	−	N/A
Session 2—Plan ahead to prevent illness	+	−	N/A
Session 3—Learn basic skills for taking care of sick children	+	−	N/A

(continued)

Reviews health manual with parent (sections 2 and 3)			
Discuss material	+	–	N/A
Answer parent's questions	+	–	N/A
Complete exercises	+	–	N/A
Demonstrate new skills	+	–	N/A
Parent practices new skills	+	–	N/A
Provide feedback to parent	+	–	N/A
Reviews what was completed during this session	+	–	N/A
Provides general feedback about session	+	–	N/A
Reminds parents to use what they have learned so far when child is ill	+	–	N/A
Asks parent to read next chapter of health manual before next mtg.	+	–	N/A
Total +			
Total + and –			
Percent correct			

Health Training Session 4
Counselor Training Checklist

Staff member _____ Date _____ Observ. # _____

\+ correct
\- incorrect

Staff member has appropriate materials ready			
True–false quiz	+	–	N/A
Health manual	+	–	N/A
Scenario cards and answer sheets	+	–	N/A
Health Recording Chart	+	–	N/A
Parent Behavior Checklist (Counselor's Version)	+	–	N/A
Doll	+	–	N/A
Health supplies	+	–	N/A
Conducts true–false quiz correctly	+	–	N/A
Conducts a "call doctor" or "treat at home/call doctor" scenario (no prompts)	+	–	N/A
Makes sure parent has all of the appropriate materials			
Health manual	+	–	N/A
Health Recording Chart	+	–	N/A
Parent Behavior Checklist (Parent's Version)	+	–	N/A
Pen or pencil	+	–	N/A
Provides positive and corrective feedback			
Provides positive, descriptive praise	+	–	N/A
Provides instructions regarding steps not correct or incomplete	+	–	N/A
Models steps as appropriate	+	–	N/A
Parent practices again steps that were incorrect or incomplete	+	–	N/A
Provides additional feedback as necessary until correct	+	–	N/A
Answers parent's questions	+	–	N/A
Provides rationale and description of remainder of session			
Recognizing when to call the doctor or seek emergency treatment	+	–	N/A
What to do when calling the doctor or seeking emergency treatment	+	–	N/A

(continued)

Reviews health manual with parent (calling the doctor and emerg. trtmt)			
Discuss material	+	–	N/A
Answer parent's questions	+	–	N/A
Complete exercises	+	–	N/A
Demonstrate new skills	+	–	N/A
Parent practices new skills	+	–	N/A
Provide feedback to parent	+	–	N/A
Provides instructions for/discussion of steps required for calling the doctor	+	–	N/A
Provides definitions of each step (see definitions)	+	–	N/A
Answers questions	+	–	N/A
Models steps for a novel "call the doctor" scenario	+	–	N/A
Has parent practice the same scenario as demonstrated	+	–	N/A
Provides positive and corrective feedback			
Provides positive, descriptive praise	+	–	N/A
Provides instructions regarding steps not correct or incomplete	+	–	N/A
Models steps as appropriate	+	–	N/A
Parent practices again steps that were incorrect or incomplete	+	–	N/A
Provides additional feedback as necessary until correct	+	–	N/A
Answers parent's questions	+	–	N/A
Provides instructions for/discussion of steps required for emergency treatment	+	–	N/A
Models steps for a novel "emergency treatment" scenario	+	–	N/A
Has parent practice the same scenario as demonstrated	+	–	N/A
Provides positive and corrective feedback			
Provides positive, descriptive praise	+	–	N/A
Provides instructions regarding steps not correct or incomplete	+	–	N/A
Models steps as appropriate	+	–	N/A
Parent practices again steps that were incorrect or incomplete	+	–	N/A
Provides additional feedback as necessary until correct	+	–	N/A
Answers parent's questions	+	–	N/A
Reviews what was completed during this session	+	–	N/A
Provides general feedback about session	+	–	N/A
Reminds parents to use what they have learned so far when child is ill	+	–	N/A
Asks parent to read next chapter of health manual before next mtg.	+	–	N/A
Explains that next session is final training session and what will be done	+	–	N/A
Total +			
Total + and –			
Percent correct			

205

References

Abidin, R. R. (1990). *Parenting Stress Index* (2nd ed.) Charlottesville, VA: Pediatric Psychology Press.

Azar, S. T., Povilaitis, T. Y., Lauretti, A. F., & Pouquette, C. L. (1998). The current status of etiological theories in intrafamilial child maltreatment. In J. R. Lutzker (Ed.), *Handbook of child abuse research and treatment* (pp. 3–30). New York: Plenum Press.

Azrin, N. H., & Besalel, V. B. (1980). *Job counselor's manual: A behavioral approach to vocational counseling.* Baltimore: University Park Press.

Beck, A. T., & Steer, R. A. (1993). *Beck Depression Inventory: Manual.* San Antonio, TX: Psychological Corporation.

Belsky, J. (1980). Child maltreatment: An ecological integration. *American Psychologist, 35,* 320–335.

Bigelow, K. M., & Lutzker, J. R. (1998). Using video to teach planned activities to parents reported for child abuse. *Child and Family Behavior Therapy, 20,* 1–14.

Bigelow, K. M., & Lutzker, J. R. (2000). Training parents at risk or reported for child abuse and neglect to identify and treat their children's illnesses. *Journal of Family Violence, 15,* 311–330.

Borck, L. E., & Fawcett, S. B. (1982). Learning counseling and problem-solving skills. New York: Haworth Press.

Campbell, R. V., O'Brien, S., Bickett, A., & Lutzker, J. R. (1983). In-home parent-training, treatment of migraine headaches, and marital counseling as an ecobehavioral approach to prevent child abuse. *Journal of Behavior Therapy and Experimental Psychiatry, 14,* 147–154.

Conners, C. K. (1990). *Conners' Rating Scales Manual.* North Tonowanda, NY: Multi-Health Systems.

Cordon, I. M., Lutzker, J. R., Bigelow, K. M., & Doctor, R. M. (1998). Evaluating Spanish protocols for teaching bonding, home safety, and health care skills to a mother reported for child abuse. *Journal of Behavior Therapy and Experimental Psychiatry, 29,* 41–54.

Delgado, L. E., & Lutzker, J. R. (1988). Training young parents to identify and report their children's illnesses. *Journal of Applied Behavior Analysis, 21,* 311–319.

DeRoma, V. M., & Hansen, D. J. (1994, November). *Development of the parental anger inventory.* Poster presented at the convention of the Association for Advancement of Behavior Therapy, San Diego, CA.

Eyberg, S., & Colvin, A. (1994, August). *Restandardization of the Eyberg Child Behavior Inventory.* Poster presented at the annual meeting of the American Psychological Association, Los Angeles.

Eyberg, S. M., & Ross, A. W. (1978). Assessment of child behavior problems: The validation of a new inventory. *Journal of Clinical Child Psychology, 7,* 113–116.

Fantuzzo, J., Weiss, A. D., & Coolahan, K. C. (1998). Community-based partnership-directed research: Actualizing community strengths to treat child victims of physical abuse and neglect. In J. R. Lutzker (Ed.), *Handbook of child abuse research and treatment* (pp. 213–238). New York: Plenum Press.

Feldman, M. A. (1998). Parents with intellectual disabilities: Implications and interventions. In J. R. Lutzker (Ed.), *Handbook of child abuse research and treatment* (pp. 401–420). New York: Plenum Press.

Fox, R. A. (1994). *Parent Behavior Checklist.* Brandon, VT: Clinical Psychology Publishing.

Fries, D. M., & Vickery, J. F. (1990). *Take care of yourself: The Healthtrac guide to medical care.* Reading, MA: Addison-Wesley.

Gershater-Molko, R. M., & Lutzker, J. R. (1999). Child neglect. In R. A. Ammerman & M. Hersen (Eds.), *Assessment of family violence: A clinical and legal sourcebook* (2nd ed., pp. 157–183). New York: Wiley.

Gershater-Molko, R. M., Lutzker, J. R., & Wesch, D. (in press). Using recidivism data to evaluate Project SafeCare: An ecobehavioral approach to teach bonding, safety, and health care skills. *Child Maltreatment.*

Greene, B. F., & Killili, S. (1998). How good does a parent have to be? Issues and examples associated with empirical assessments of parenting adequacy in cases of child abuse and neglect. In J. R. Lutzker (Ed.), *Handbook of child abuse research and treatment* (pp. 53–72). New York: Plenum Press.

Hansen, D. J., & MacMillan, V. M. (1990). Behavioral assessment of child abusive and neglectful families: Recent developments and current issues. *Behavior Modification, 14,* 255–278.

Hansen, D. J., Warner-Rogers, J. E., & Hecht, D. B. (1998). Implementing and evaluating an individualized behavioral intervention program for maltreating families: Clinical and research issues. In J. R. Lutzker (Ed.). *Handbook of child abuse research and treatment* (pp. 75–116). New York: Plenum Press.

Hoffman-Plotkin, D., & Twentyman, C. T. (1984). A multimodal assessment of behavioral and cognitive deficits in abused and neglected preschoolers. *Child Development, 55,* 794–802.

Huynen, K. B., Lutzker, J. R., Bigelow, K. M., Touchette, P. E., & Campbell, R. V. (1996). Planned activities training for mothers with children with developmental disabilities: Community generalization and follow-up. *Behavior Modification, 20,* 406–427.

Kapitanoff, S., Lutzker, J. R., & Bigelow, K. M. (2000). Cultural issues in the relation between child disabilities and child abuse. *Aggression and Violent Behavior, 5,* 227–244.

Kazdin, A. E. (1982). *Single-case research designs: Methods for clinical and applied settings.* New York: Oxford University Press.

Kempe, C., Silverman, F., Steele, B., Droegemueller, W., & Silver, H. (1962). The battered child syndrome. *Journal of the American Medical Association, 181,* 17–24.

Loyd, B. H., & Abidin, R. R. (1985). Revision of the Parenting Stress Index. *Journal of Pediatric Psychology, 10,* 169–177.

Lutzker, J. R. (1994). Aspectos practicos de la prestacion de servicios ecoconductuales de amplio espectro a familias (Practical issues in delivering broad-based ecobehavioral services to families). *Revista Mexicana de Psicologia, 11,* 87–96.

Lutzker, J. R. (1998). Child abuse and neglect: Weaving theory, research and treatment in the Twenty-first century. In J. R. Lutzker (Ed.), *Handbook of child abuse research and treatment* (pp. 563–570). New York: Plenum Press.

Lutzker, J. R. (2000). Balancing research and treatment in child maltreatment: The quest for good data and practical service. In D. J. Hansen (Ed.), *Nebraska Symposium on Motivation: Vol. 43. Motivation and child maltreatment* (pp. 221–224). Lincoln: University of Nebraska Press.

Lutzker, J. R., Bigelow, K. M., Doctor, R. M., Gershater, R. M., & Greene, B. F. (1998). An ecobehavioral model for the prevention and treatment of child abuse and neglect: History and applications. In J. R. Lutzker (Ed.), *Handbook of child abuse research and treatment* (pp. 239–266). New York: Plenum Press.

Lutzker, J. R., Bigelow, K. M., Swensen, C. C., Doctor, R. M., & Kessler, M. L. (1999). Problems related to child abuse and neglect. In S. D. Netherton, D. Holmes, & C. E. Walker (Eds.), *Child and adolescent psychological disorders* (pp. 520–548). New York: Oxford University Press.

Lutzker, J. R., Frame, R. E., & Rice, J. M. (1982). Project 12–Ways: An ecobehavioral approach to the treatment and prevention of child abuse and neglect. *Education and Treatment of Children, 5,* 141–155.

Lutzker, J. R., & Rice, J. M. (1987). Using recidivism data to evaluate Project 12–Ways: An ecobehavioral approach to the treatment and prevention of child abuse and neglect. *Journal of Family Violence, 2,* 283–290.

MacMillan, V. M., Guevremont, D. C., & Hansen, D. J. (1988). Problem-solving training with a multiply distressed abusive and neglectful mother: Effects on social insularity, negative affect, and stress. *Journal of Family Violence, 3,* 313–326.

Mandel, U., Bigelow, K. M., & Lutzker, J. R. (1998). Using video to reduce home safety hazards with parents reported for child abuse or neglect. *Journal of Family Violence, 13,* 147–162.

McGimsey, J. F., Lutzker, J. R., & Greene, B. F. (1994). Validating and teaching affective adult–child interaction skills. *Behavior Modification, 18,* 209–224.

Metchikian, K. L., Mink, J. M., Bigelow, K. M., Lutzker, J. R., & Doctor, R. M. (1999). Reducing home safety hazards in the homes of parents reported for neglect. *Child and Family Behavior Therapy, 3,* 23–34.

Milner, J. S. (1986). *The Child Abuse Potential Inventory Manual* (2nd ed.). Webster, NC: Psytec.

Milner, J. S. (1994). Assessing physical child abuse risk: The Child Abuse Potential Inventory. *Clinical Psychology Review, 14,* 547–583.

Milner, J. S., Murphy, W. D., Valle, L. A., & Toliver, R. M. (1999). Assessment issues in child abuse evaluations. In J. R. Lutzker (Ed.), *Handbook of child abuse research and treatment* (pp. 75–115). New York: Plenum.

National Center on Child Abuse and Neglect. (1993). *Study findings: National study of the incidence and severity of child abuse and neglect.* Washington, DC: U.S. Government Printing Office.

National Research Council. (1993). *Understanding child abuse and neglect.* Washington, DC: National Academy Press.

National Safety Council. (2000). *Injury facts.* Chicago: National Safety Council.

O'Brien, M. P., Lutzker, J. R., & Campbell, R. V. (1993). Consumer evaluation of an ecobehavioral program for families with children with developmental disabilities. *Journal of Mental Health Administration, 20*(3), 278–284.

Peterson, L., & Gable, S. (1998). Holistic injury prevention. In J. R. Lutzker (Ed.), *Handbook of child abuse research and treatment* (pp. 291–318). New York: Plenum Press.

Pittman, A., Wolfe, D. A., & Wekerle, C. (1998). Prevention during adolescence: The youth relationships project. In J. R. Lutzker (Ed.), Handbook of child abuse research and treatment (pp. 341–356). New York: Plenum Press.

Poppen, R. (1988). *Behavioral relaxation training.* New York: Pergamon Press.

Portwood, S. G., Reppucci, N. D., & Mitchell, M. S. (1998). Balancing rights and responsibilities: Legal perspectives on child maltreatment. In J. R. Lutzker (Ed.), *Handbook of child abuse research and treatment* (pp. 31–52). New York: Plenum Press.

Sanders, M. R., & Dadds, M. R. (1982). The effects of planned activities and child management procedures on parent training: An analysis of setting generality. *Behavior Therapy, 13,* 452–461.

Sanders, M. R., & Dadds, M. R. (1993). *Behavioral family interventions.* Boston: Allyn & Bacon.

Solis, M. L., & Abidin, R. R. (1991). The Spanish version Parenting Stress Index: A psychometric study. *Journal of Clinical Child Psychology, 20,* 372–378.

Stoppard, M. (1986). *Baby and child A to Z medical handbook.* New York: Body Press/Perigee Books.

Striefel, S., Robinson, M. A., & Truhn, P. (1998). Dealing with child abuse and neglect within a comprehensive family-support program. In J. R. Lutzker (Ed.), *Handbook of child abuse research and treatment* (pp. 267–290). New York: Plenum Press.

Tertinger, D. A., Greene, B. F., & Lutzker, J. R. (1984). Home safety: Development and validation of one component of an ecobehavioral treatment program for abused and neglected children. *Journal of Applied Behavior Analysis, 17,* 159–174.

Tymchuk, A. J. (1998). The importance of matching educational interventions to parent needs in child maltreatment: Issues, methods, and recommendations. In J. R. Lutzker (Ed.), *Handbook of child abuse research and treatment* (pp. 421–448). New York: Plenum Press.

U.S. Department of Health and Human Services, National Center on Child Abuse and Neglect (1995). *Child maltreatment, 1993: Reports from the states to the National Center on Child Abuse and Neglect.* Washington, DC: U.S. Government Printing Office.

Watson-Perczel, M., Lutzker, J. R., Greene, B. F., & McGimpsey, B. J. (1988). Assessment and modification of home cleanliness among families adjudicated for child neglect. *Behavior Modification, 12,* 57–81.

Wesch, D., & Lutzker, J. R. (1991). A comprehensive evaluation of Project 12–Ways: An ecobehavioral program for treating and preventing child abuse and neglect. *Journal of Family Violence, 6,* 17–35.

Wolf, M. M. (1978). Social validity: The case for subjective measurement or how applied behavior analysis is finding its heart. *Journal of Applied Behavior Analysis, 11,* 203–214.

Wolfe, D. A. (1987). *Child abuse: Implications for child development and psychopathology.* Newbury Park, CA: Sage.

Wolfe, D. A. (1999). *Child abuse: Implications for child development and psychopathology* (2nd ed.). Newbury Park, CA: Sage.

Yung, B. R., & Hammond, W. R. (1998). Breaking the cycle: A culturally sensitive violence prevention program for African-American children and adolescents. In J. R. Lutzker (Ed.), *Handbook of child abuse research and treatment* (pp. 319–340). New York: Plenum Press.

Author Index

Subject Index

(Page numbers in bold indicate copies of forms available in appendices.)